Dodging Bullets: Surviving Breast Cancer

An Intimate Look at My Mayo Clinic Breast Cancer Experience

By Linda Hanson

Front Cover: Sitting by spring tulips at the Mayo Clinic's downtown campus in Rochester, Minnesota.

Back Cover: Standing by Mayo Clinic's "150 Year's of Serving Humanity" semi, traveling exhibit at the Mayo Clinic's Peace Plaza in downtown Rochester. The exhibit went on to travel more than 18,000 miles to 40 cities across the U.S. and Canada.

ISBN-13: 978-1508966395

ISBN-10: 1508966397

Introduction

Doctoring at the Mayo Clinic was not originally planned. Originally, the plan was to do all of my doctoring in northern Minnesota. Following my third surgery in Fosston, Minnesota, my surgeon sent me to Fargo, North Dakota to meet with an oncologist (cancer doctor). To my surprise, the oncologist in Fargo had a completely different set of opinions from my surgeon. The oncologists exam left me feeling violated. I left feeling so down-and-discouraged that I felt that I'd rather take my chances by skipping treatments altogether, before going through what he had in-store for me. Little did I know at the time that this experience was a blessing in disguise for guiding me to the Mayo Clinic.

Upon notifying my surgeon to share my experience, he reassured me that they would do anything for me. So I asked to be recommended to the Mayo Clinic. It must have been meant to be, because during my first appointment, I ran into a friend from back home in the waiting room. This friend shared her breast cancer story of doing all of her doctoring at the Mayo Clinic, and highly encouraged me to do the same.

Sixteen chemotherapy treatments, thirty radiation treatments, one-month of physical therapy, and I'm cancer free!

Timeline

July 22, 2013
Had mammogram.

August 20, 2013
Received news that the lump was malignant, Stage 3 Aggressive Breast Cancer.

August 21, 2013
First surgery (out-patient) to remove five-centimeter lump in Fosston, Minnesota.
Tumor was the size of a golf ball or larger.

September 18, 2013
Second surgery to take a biopsy of the right breast in Fosston.
Sentinel Lymph Node was also removed.

November 13, 2013
Third surgery (out-patient) in Fosston to clean-up margins around where the cancerous tumors had been present.

January 13, 2014 - June 2, 2014
Sixteen weekly chemotherapy treatments.
Twelve Taxol Chemotherapy & Four E.C. Chemotherapy treatments.

February 10, 2014 - February 12, 2014
Hospitalized with Pulmonary Embolism Blood Clots.

June 9, 2014
Ultrasound of breast.
Good news: "No cancer in lymph nodes."

June 23, 2014 - August 4, 2014
Six weeks of thirty radiation treatments.

Attitude

Maintaining a positive attitude is critical to getting through cancer treatments. Keep in mind how advancements in recent years has made it possible to view cancer as more of a temporary condition, where once you complete your treatments, you will go on to live a long, healthy, cancer-free life.

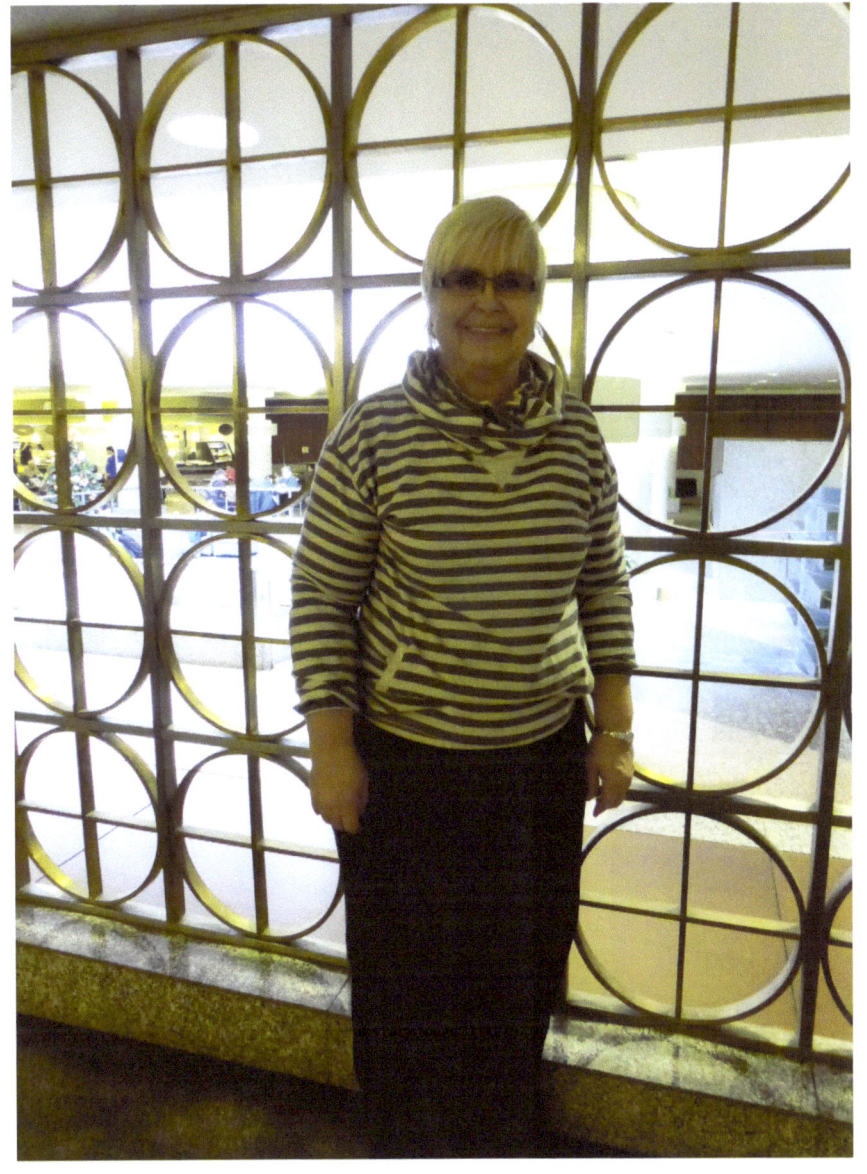

First Chemotherapy (Taxol) Treatment.
January 13, 2014

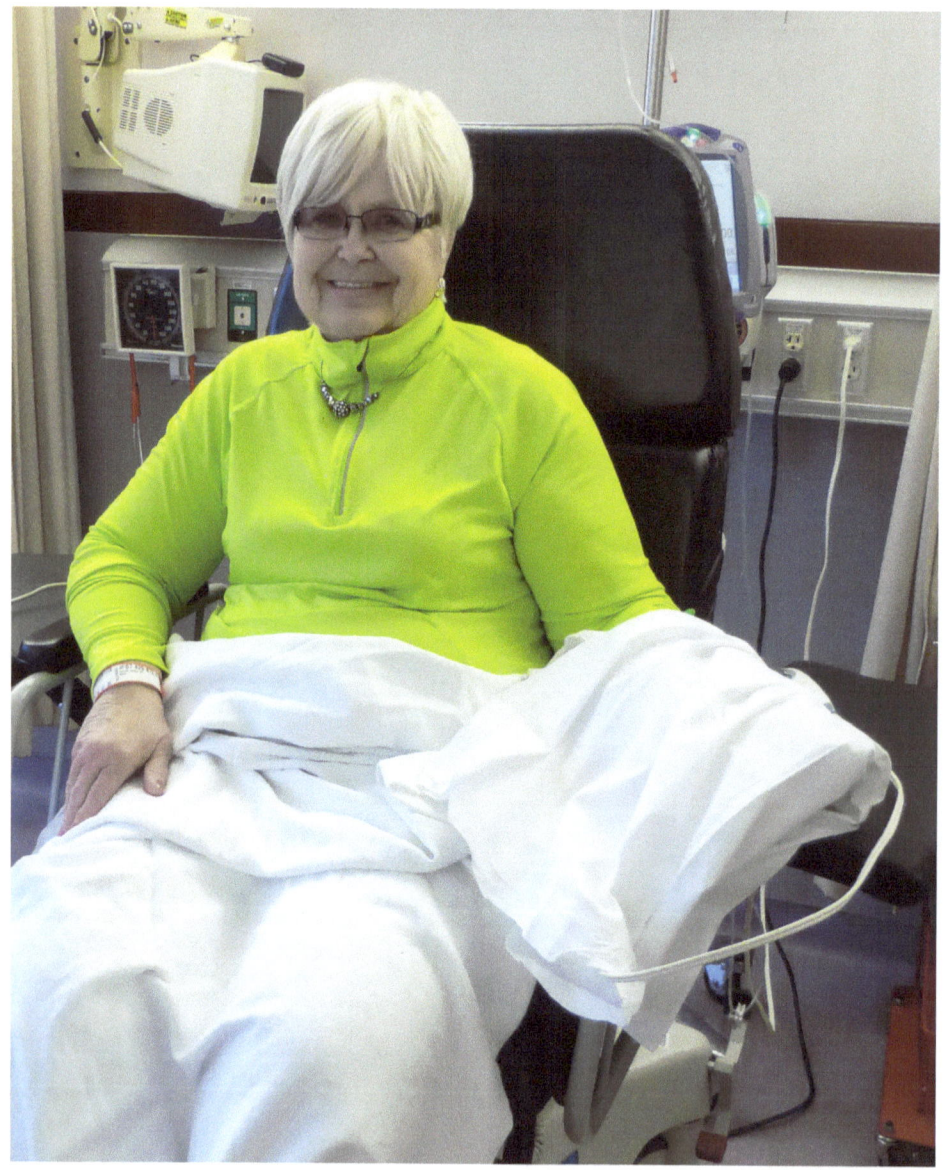

No Port Required

A heating pad was placed on my hand for about five minutes before each chemotherapy treatment to make it easier to insert the IV tube in a vein.

The Mayo Clinic is not like so many medical facilities that may offer no option but to surgically insert a "port" catheter in their cancer patients. Port's require additional care of cleaning, draining, and needing to be surgically removed. What a relief that the Mayo Clinic administers chemotherapy without requiring a port.

Second Chemotherapy (Taxol) Treatment.

January 20, 2014

Snacks

One of the nice perks during chemotherapy treatments are the snacks. Orange juice, pretzels, and cookies are among my favorites.

The IV's are connected to mobile equipment that allows you to get up and use nearby restrooms during each three hour treatment.

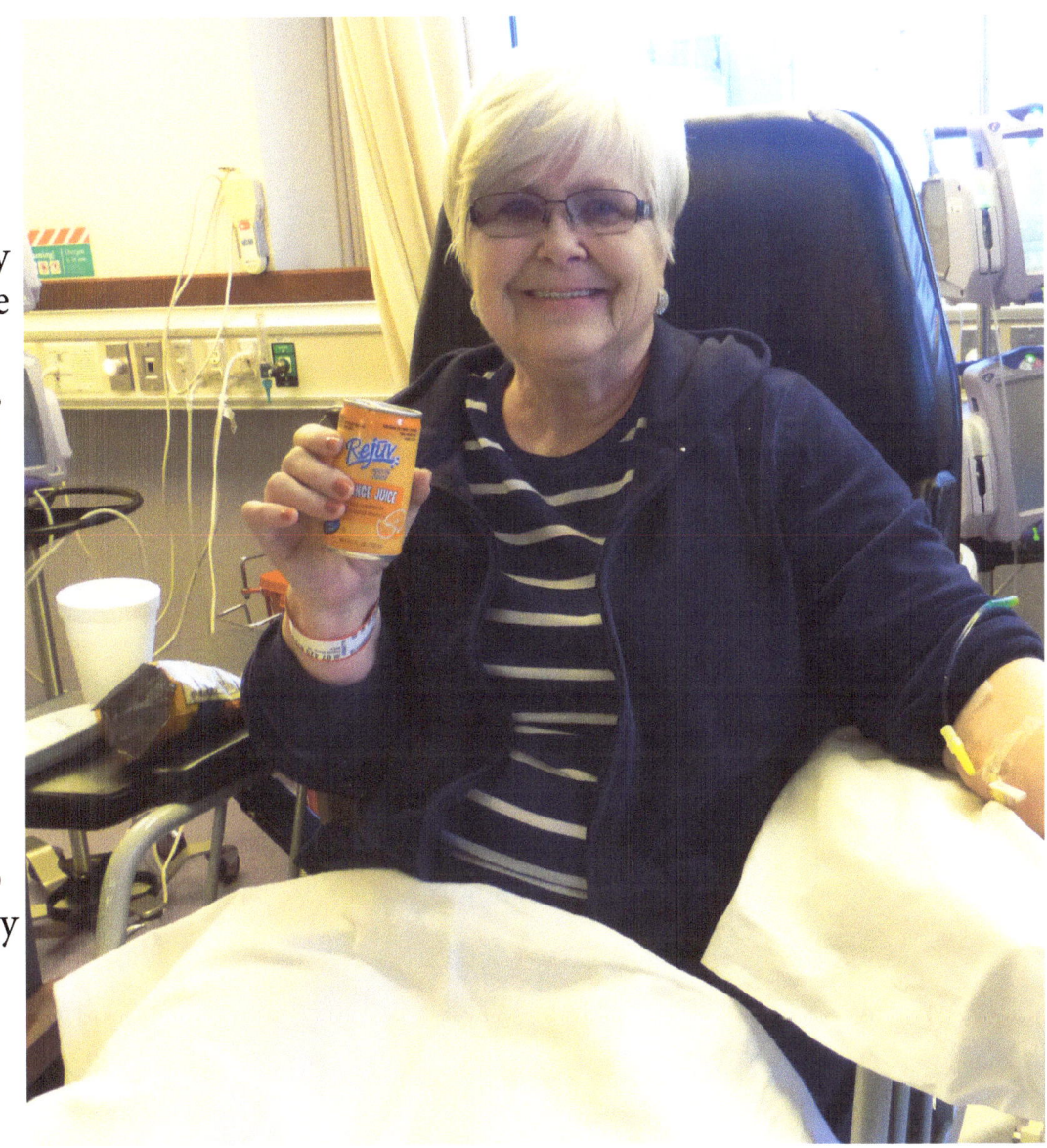

Third Chemotherapy (Taxol) Treatment.
January 28, 2014

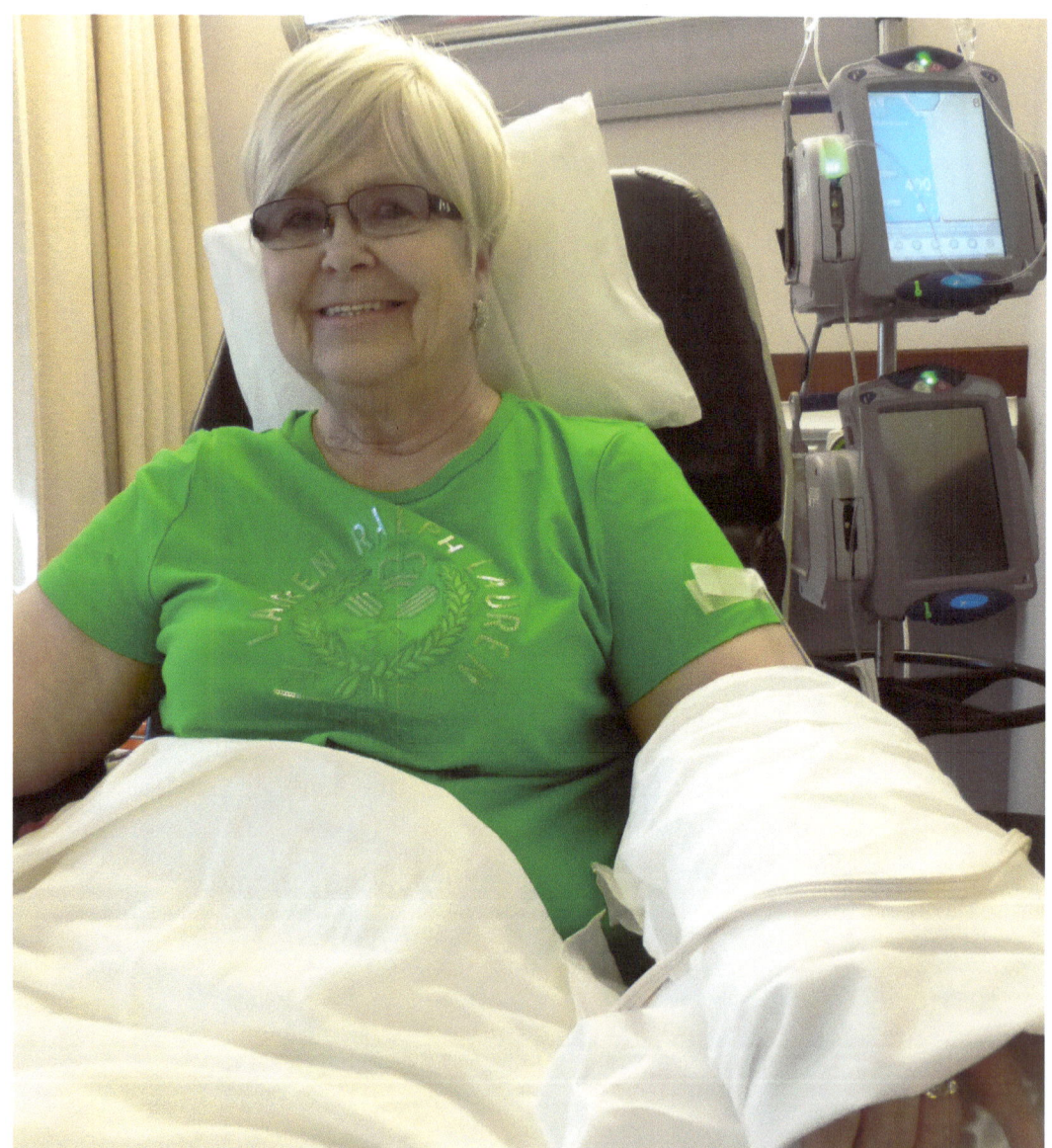

Outlook

Everybody always thinks you get so sick from chemo. It doesn't have to be like that. We all are different. Just keep telling yourself that you won't get sick and that it's nothing. It works!

Fourth Chemotherapy (Taxol) Treatment.
February 3, 2014

Dodging Bullets

A team of six doctors came into my room, stood in a semi-circle around my bed, and told me how lucky I was to survive the "blood clots" (Pulmonary Embolisms), caused by the reaction between the chemotherapy and cancer. They said that I was "Dodging Bullets" and that very few survive what I experienced.

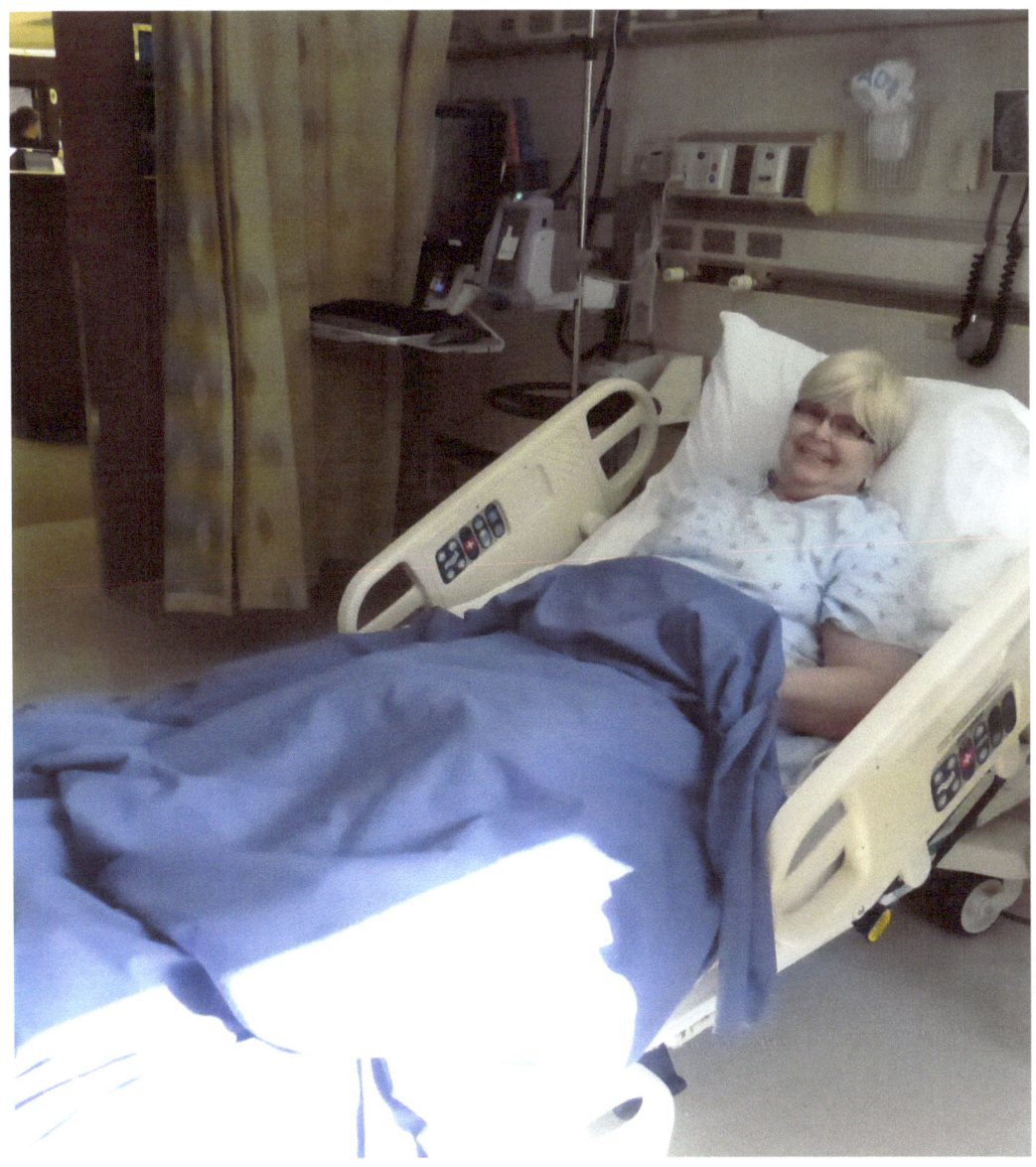

Admitted to Mayo Methodist Hospital with Pulmonary Embolism (P.E.) blood clots in both lungs.
February 10 - 12, 2014

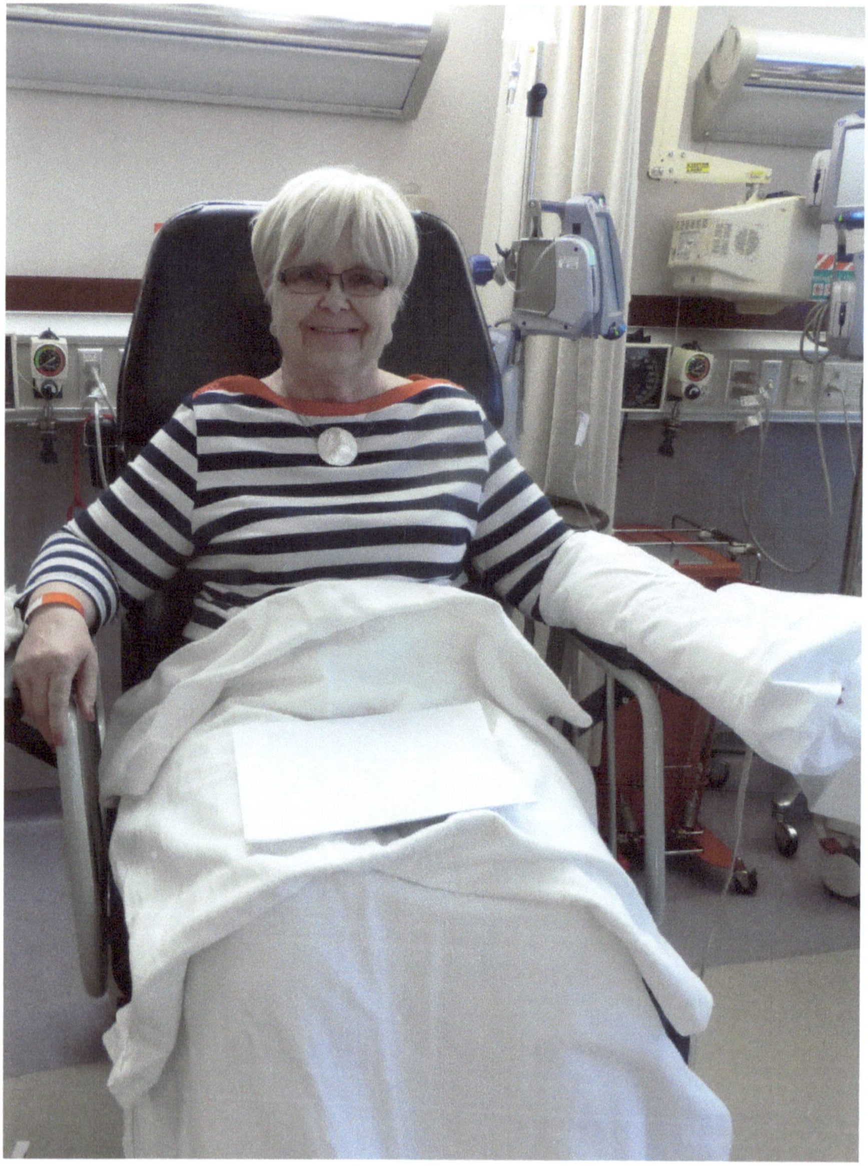

Breast Cancer Mentors

Breast cancer survivors volunteer their time to visit with current breast cancer patients to speak about the social aspects of breast cancer and to share their breast cancer experiences.

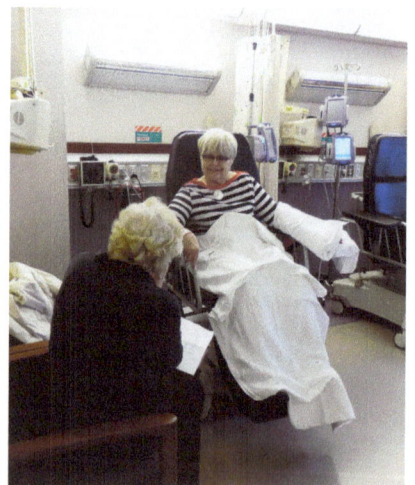

Fifth Chemotherapy (Taxol) Treatment.
February 24, 2014

Routine

The routine each week for sixteen weeks of chemotherapy included driving seven hours from northern Minnesota to the Mayo Clinic. Leaving home at 11 p.m. and driving all night, made it possible to get to the Mayo Clinic for Monday morning appointments. Most of the time, we would drive home after my treatments, for a total of fourteen hours of driving in a single day. It became normal to nap in waiting rooms and the car when we arrived at the Mayo Clinic early.

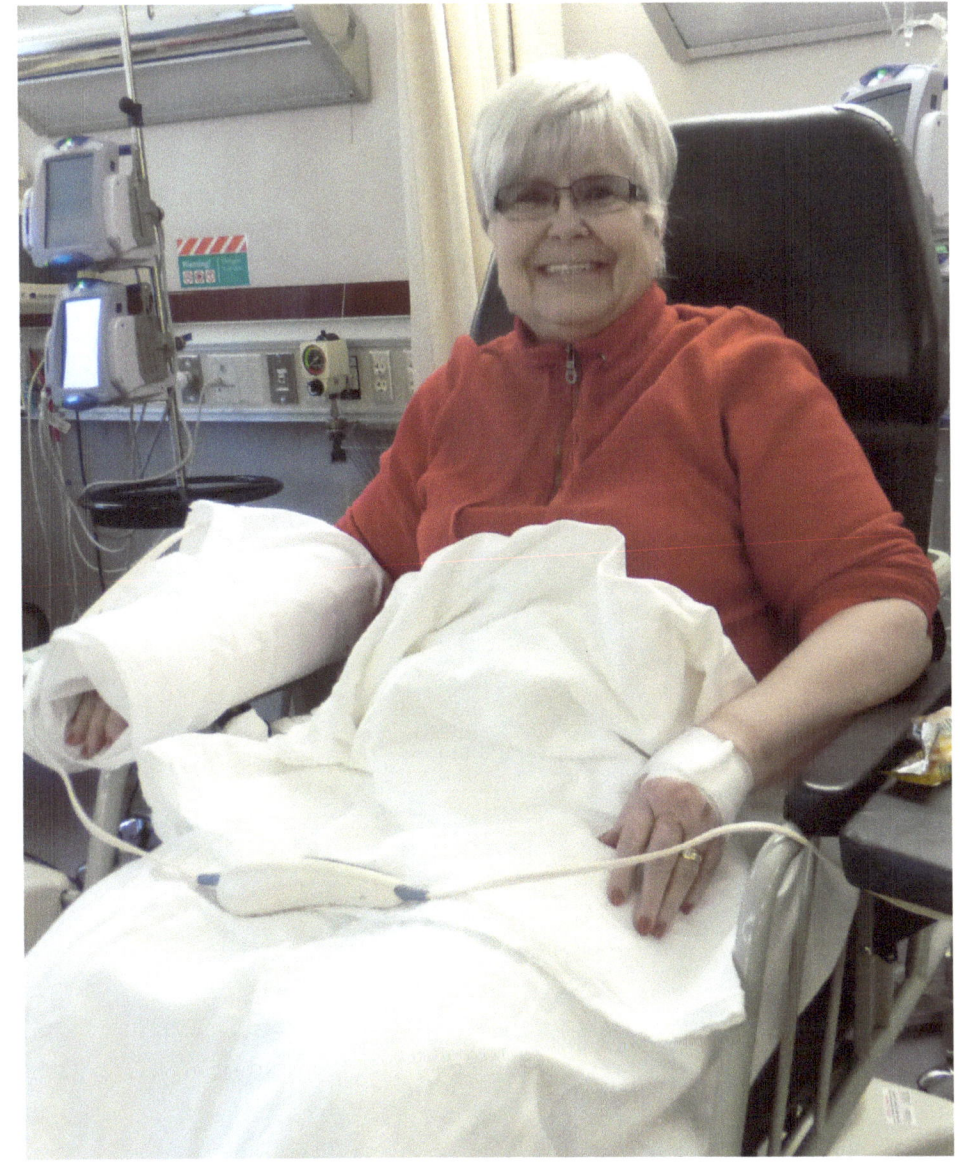

Sixth Chemotherapy (Taxol) Treatment.
March 3, 2014

Quality Of Care

On paper, chemotherapy treatments at the Mayo Clinic may sound similar or even identical to what other medical facilities up north would offer. But the way the treatments are given can be a world apart. Some options that appeared to be a convenience to me at face value, just wasn't worth it. The option to take less, but more potent treatments every two or three weeks was presented to me. My doctor highly suggested the less potent, weekly treatments. These treatments were effective and I didn't get sick. Out of meeting with dozens of medical professionals at the Mayo Clinic, only a few mentioned having my treatments up north. Doing all of your doctoring at the Mayo Clinic is worth pursuing, especially when dealing with serious medical conditions.

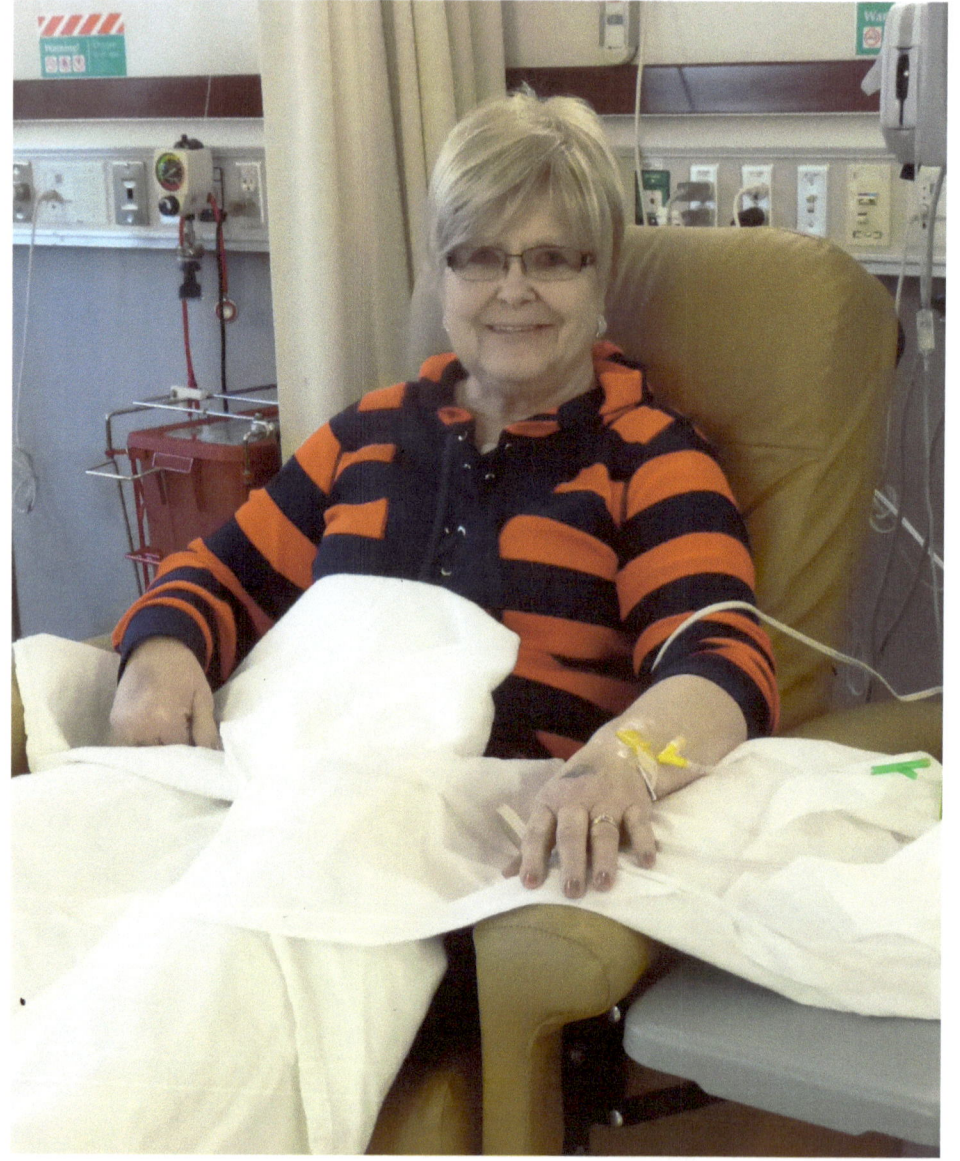

Seventh Chemotherapy (Taxol) Treatment.
March 10, 2014

Blood Clots

Anticoagulant medicine to treat blood clots in cancer patients is different from the Warfarin/Coumadin medicine that is given to non-cancer patients in-order to prevent internal bleeding. I was shown how to give myself pre-loaded shots of Lovenox in my stomach twice a day for a few months. I never dreamed that I could do it, but there was nothing to it. Lovenox is an expensive medicine, so I switched to an oral Xeralto pill. Both Lovenox and Xeralto dissolve existing blood clots and prevent new blood clots from forming, without causing internal bleeding.

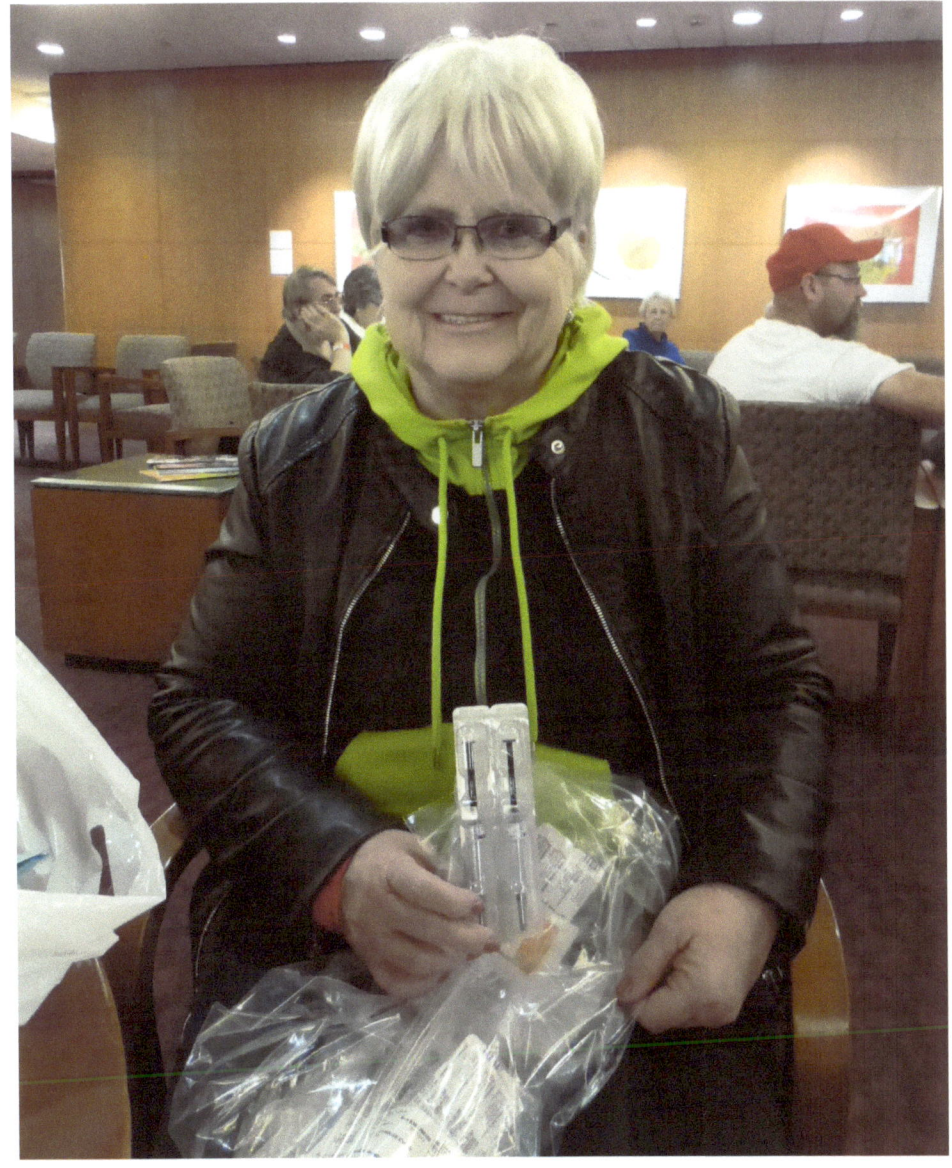

Lovenox (Heparin) Syringes for Pulmonary Embolisms (P.E.'s).

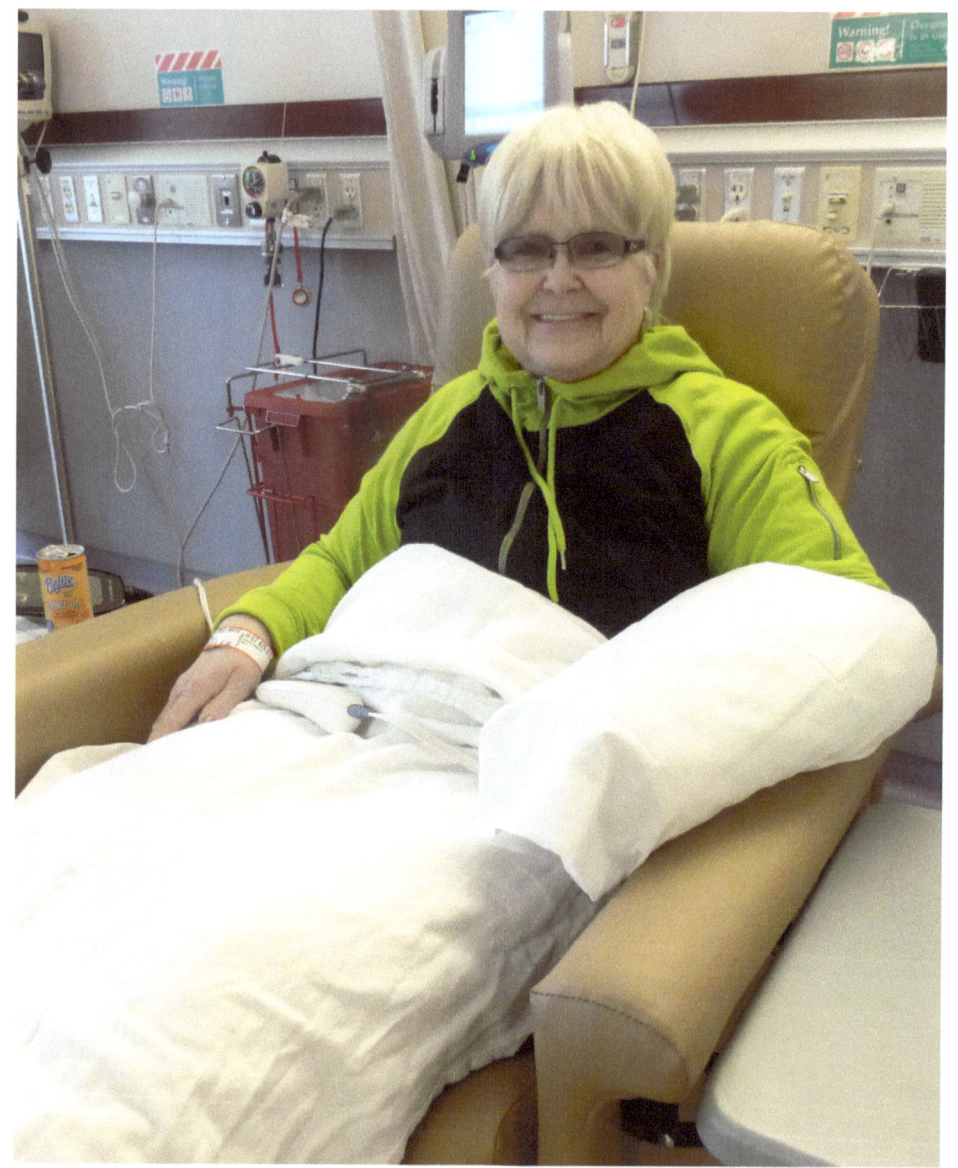

The Doctors

When you meet with a doctor at the Mayo Clinic, a team of perhaps half-a-dozen doctors are working together on your case behind the scenes. My doctor would also keep tabs on my blood count levels and overall health, even when I was not meeting with that doctor each week. The compassionate care that you receive at the Mayo Clinic truly makes it clear that you are truly treated as an individual and not a number. What's impressive is how even the most common of medical patients are treated with the same dignity and respect as the kings, queens, and celebrities who doctor at the Mayo Clinic.

Eighth Chemotherapy (Taxol) Treatment.
March 17, 2014

Volunteers

Some volunteers offer free hand massages, while you receive your chemo treatment. Volunteers at the Mayo Clinic wear blue jackets and offer a variety of hospitality, from those who stand throughout the clinic to offer directions to volunteers who are more than happy to bring you coffee, juice, water, and snacks during your treatments. After just a couple of treatments, volunteers become familiar faces, who welcome conversation, and offer their love and support to folks who find themselves in unfamiliar territory.

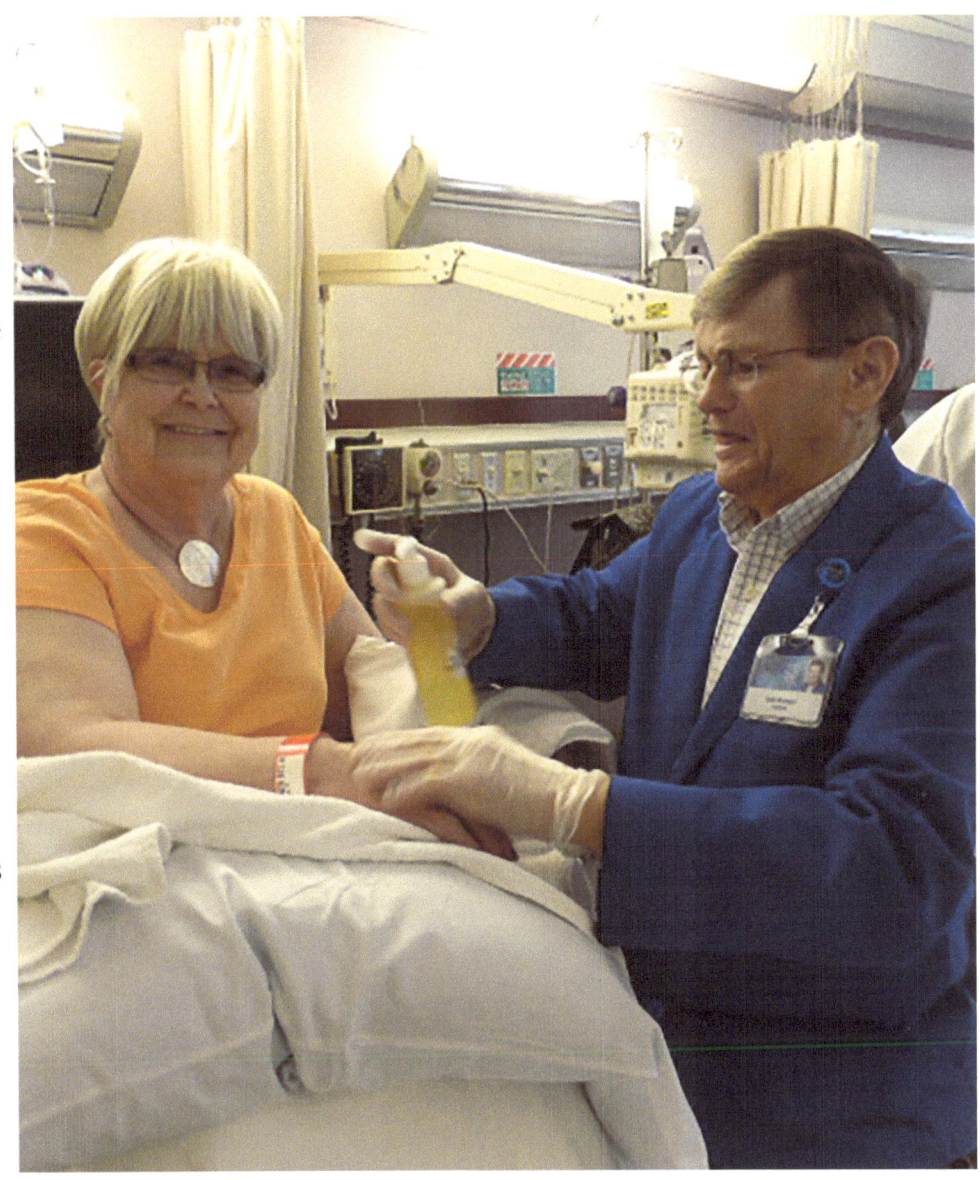

Ninth Chemotherapy (Taxol) Treatment.
March 24, 2014

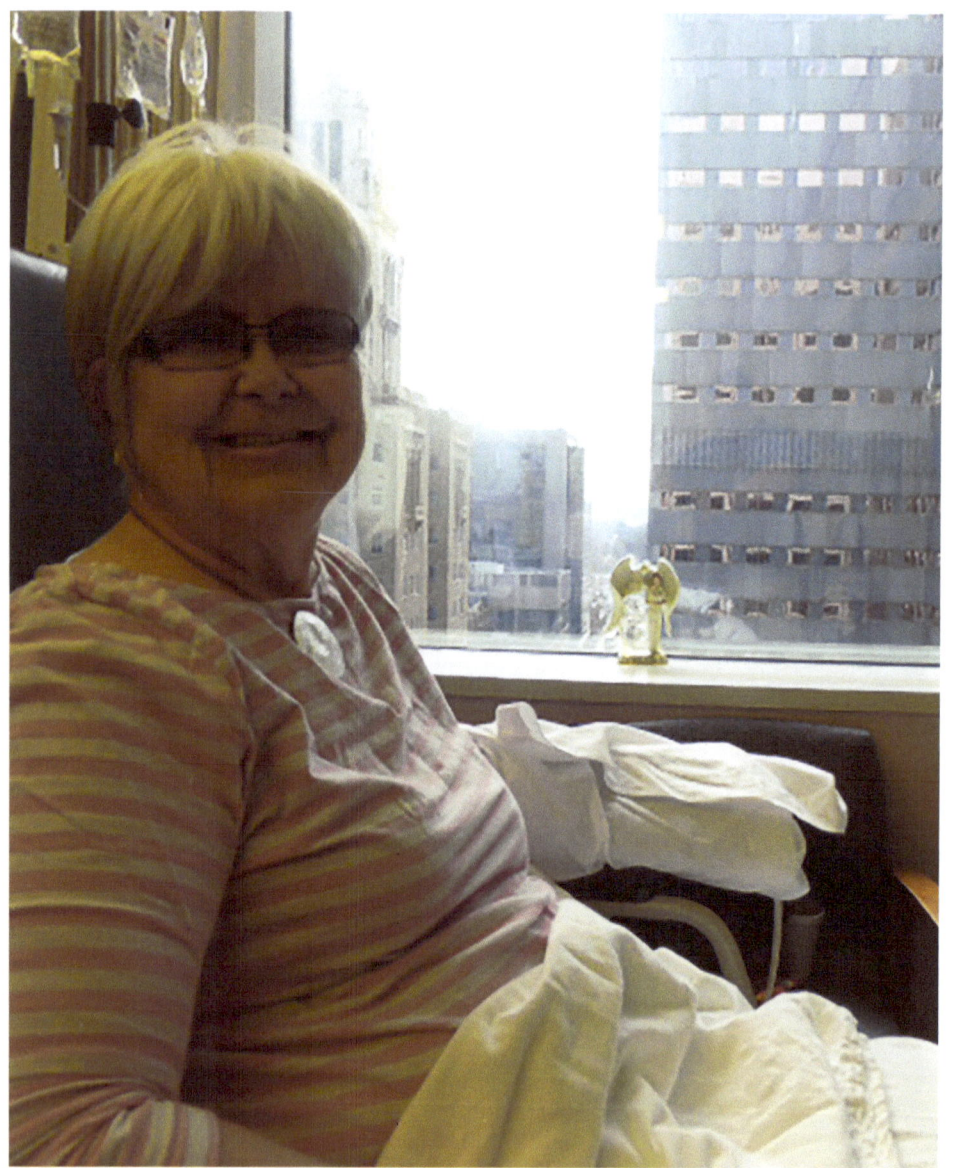

Power of Prayer

I prayed really hard and asked the Lord to be with me every step of the way to hold my hand and walk me through this. From the day I received the call from my doctor that the results of my lumpectomy was malignant, I never was worried. I just knew that I would be OK. It was like I was told, "Do not worry. It will be fine. I will be with you and help you through this." I guess that is what got me through it. I felt so relaxed and calm about it. I was happy that I did not need a port. I was expecting it. My doctor at the Mayo said, "We do not do that here, you will not need that." I couldn't believe how nice that went for me.

Tenth Chemotherapy (Taxol) Treatment.
March 31, 2014

Side-Effects

I do have to admit, my legs became weak. I've been trying to exercise my legs by getting outside to walk. That has helped a lot. I am hoping to keep up walking and lose weight to strengthen my legs. Several months after completing chemotherapy and radiation, I am losing some toe nails. The toe nails become loose and fall off. I don't even feel it. It just feels like a small stone in my sock and when I take my sock off, here is a toe nail.

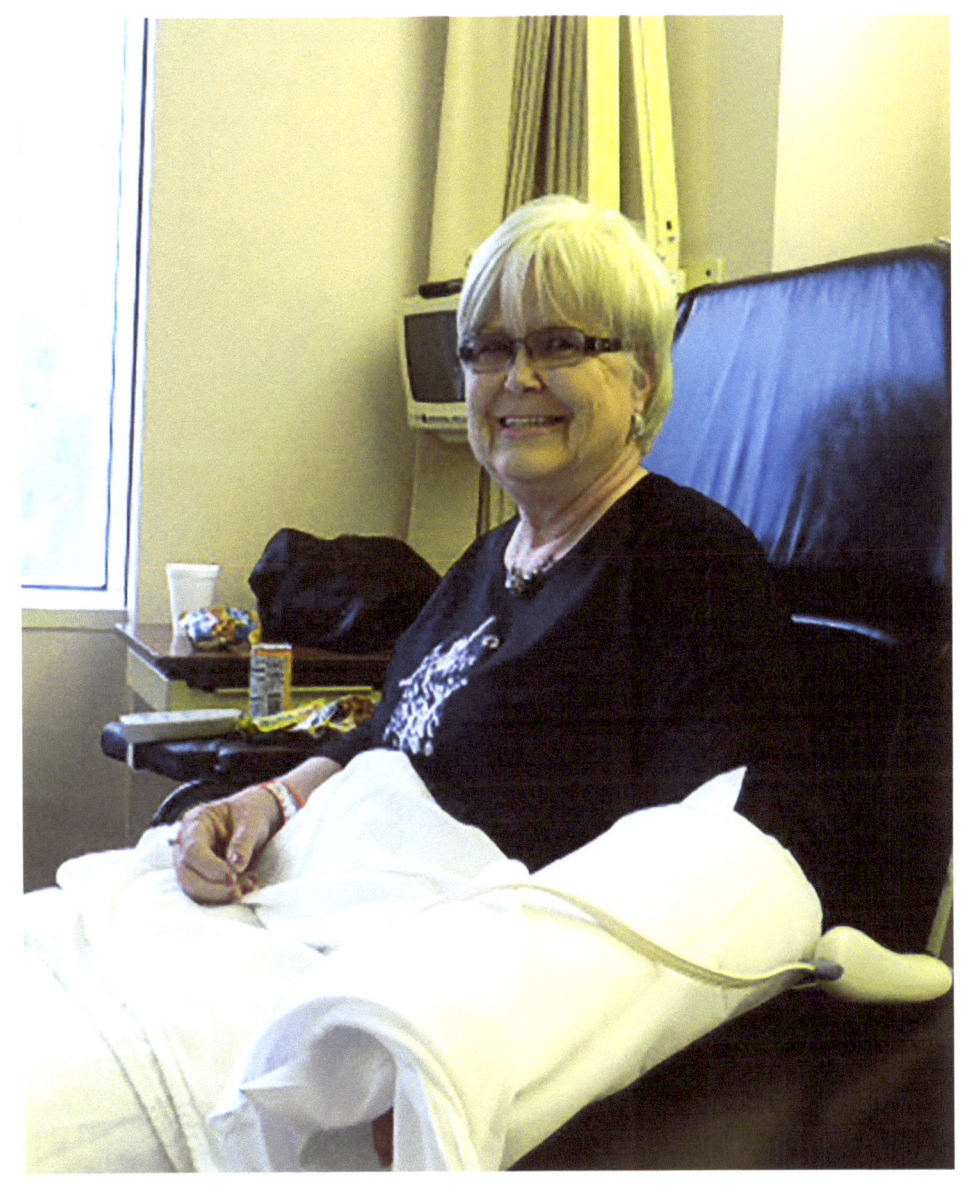

Eleventh Chemotherapy (Taxol) Treatment.
April 7, 2014

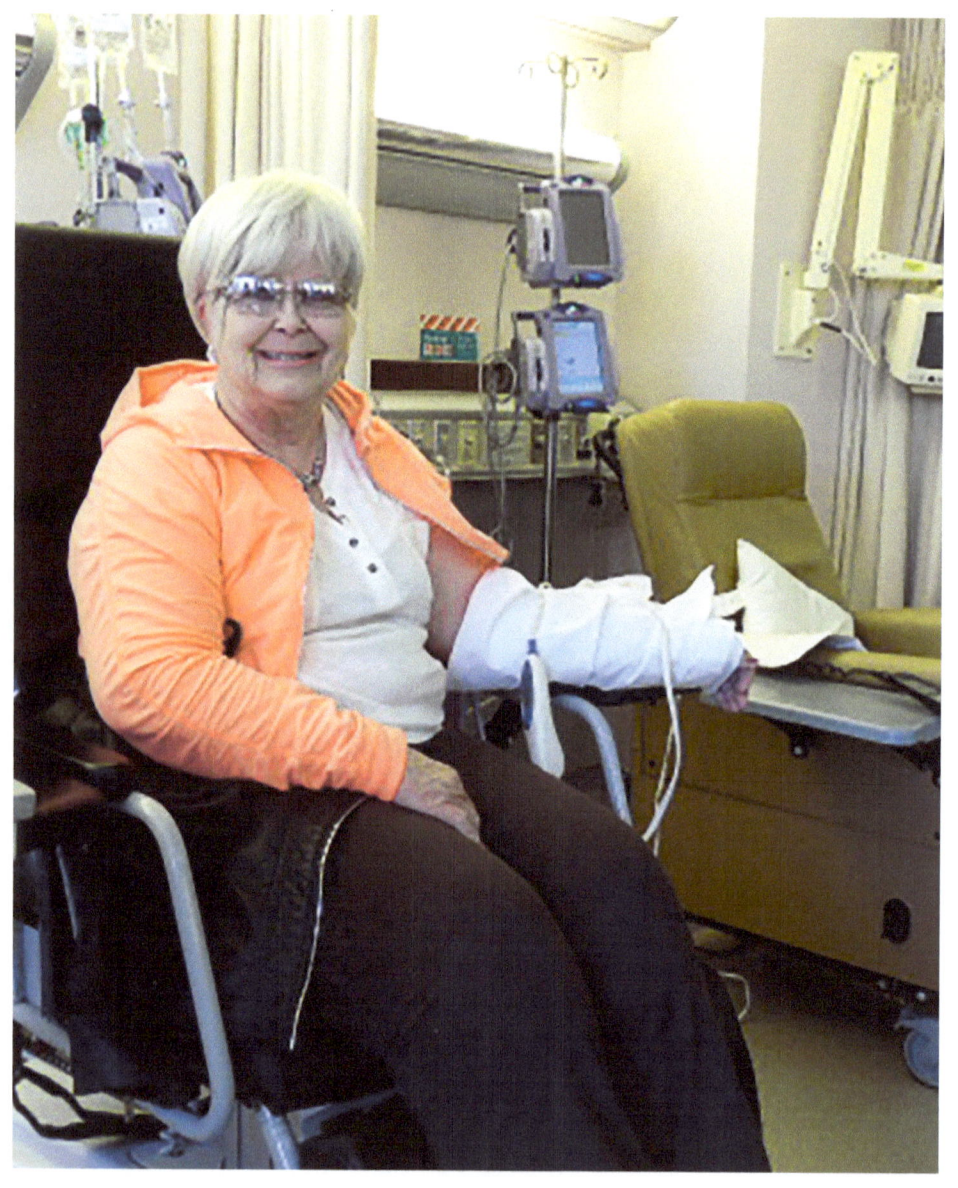

Importance of Support Advocates

If at all possible, have an advocate along to your appointments. Advocates go back with you to your medical appointments to meet with doctors for support, take notes, ask questions, speak-up if concerns arise, drive, run errands, research topics discussed with your doctors, and may even push you in a wheel-chair if needed. My son traveled with me as an advocate.

Twelfth Chemotherapy (Taxol) Treatment.
April 14, 2014

Pre-Meds

Three different pre-meds were given to me to prepare my system for each Taxol chemotherapy treatment. These pre-meds made me feel better than before each treatment. This good effect lasted for three or four days.

Each pre-med took fifteen minutes to run into my system. The Taxol chemotherapy took an hour. Each treatment lasted about three hours.

The Mayo Clinic mixes up the chemotherapy medicine fresh, after you are seated for your treatment.

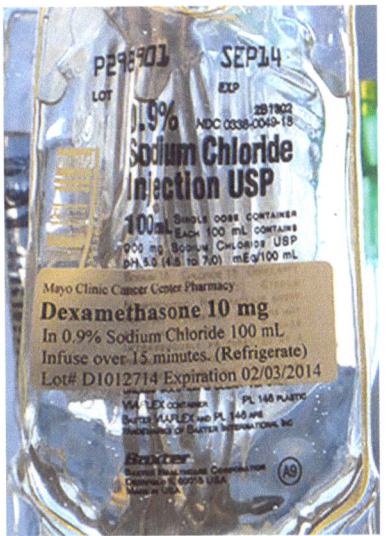

Dexamethasone (Steroid)
First Taxol Pre-Med.

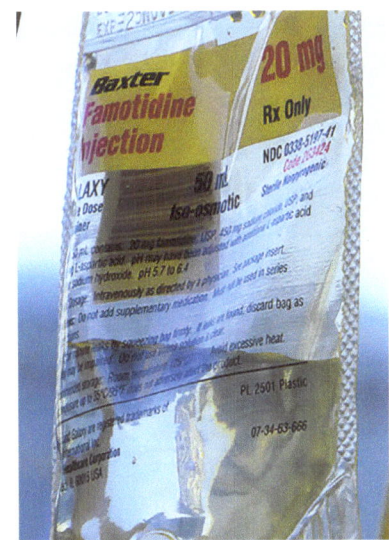

Pepcid (Antihistamine)
Second Taxol Pre-Med.

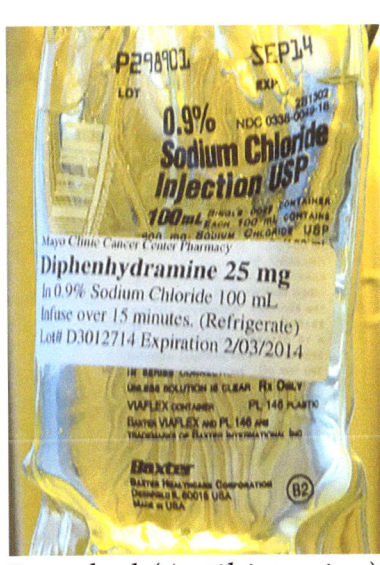

Benadryl (Antihistamine)
Third Taxol Pre-Med.

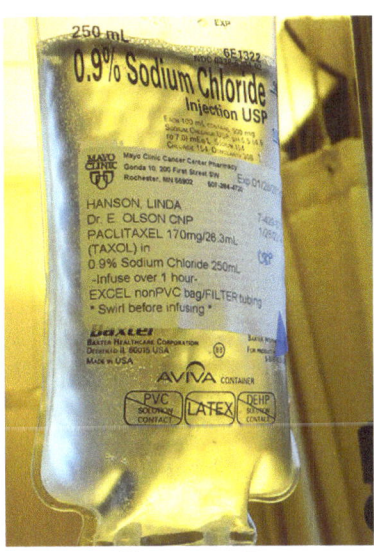

Taxol
Chemotherapy

Taxol Chemotherapy Pre-Meds

Popsicles

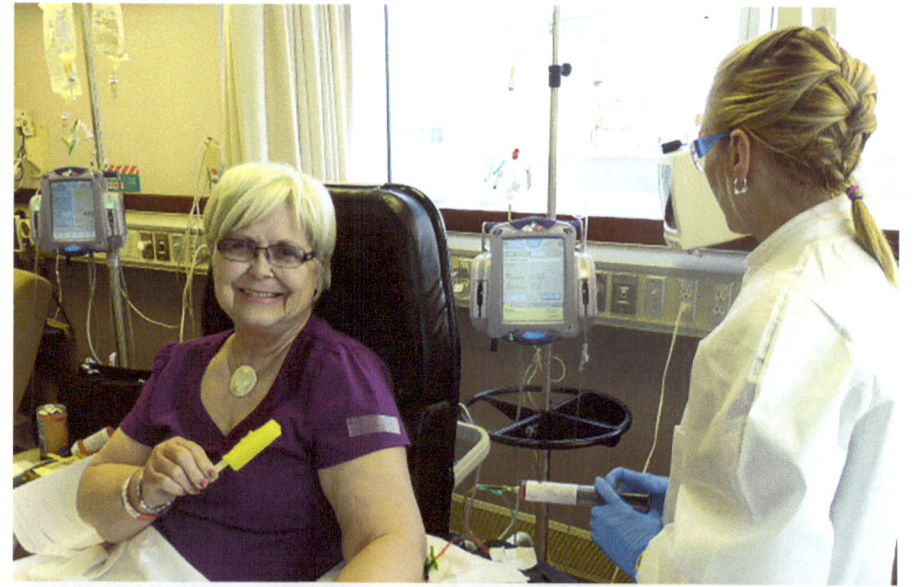

The last four chemotherapy treatments were a different type of chemotherapy. A nurse slowly pushed three different syringes of a red fluid into my veins, while I sucked on popsicles to prevent mouth sores from instantly forming in my mouth. During these treatments an IV of saline solution was also run into my system.

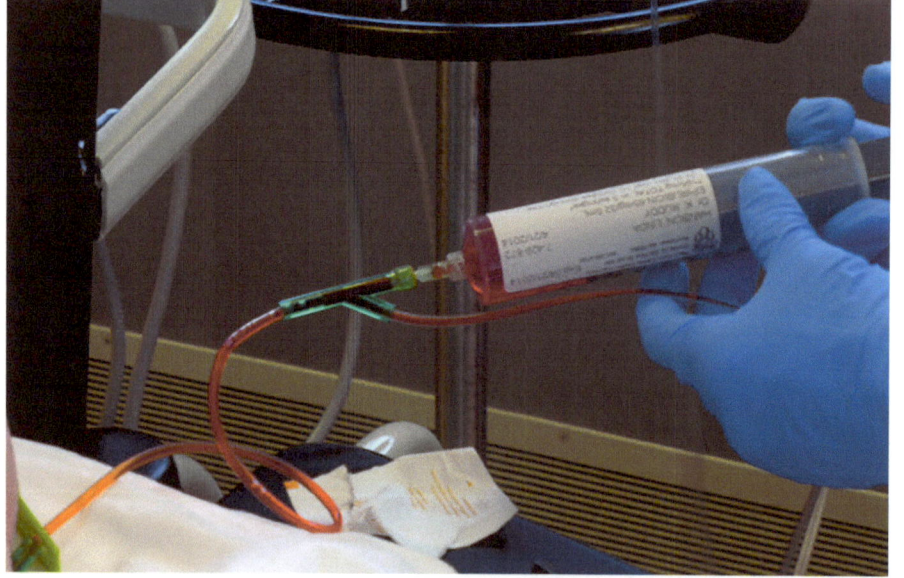

First E.C. (Epirubicin Cyclophosphamide) Chemotherapy Treatment. | April 21, 2014
Neulasta Booster Shot | April 22, 2014

Feeling Comfortable With Your Doctors & Nurses

A great sense of comfort came from experiencing the compassionate care at the Mayo Clinic. If you do not feel completely comfortable with your doctor(s) or nurse(s), do not hesitate seeking a second opinion.

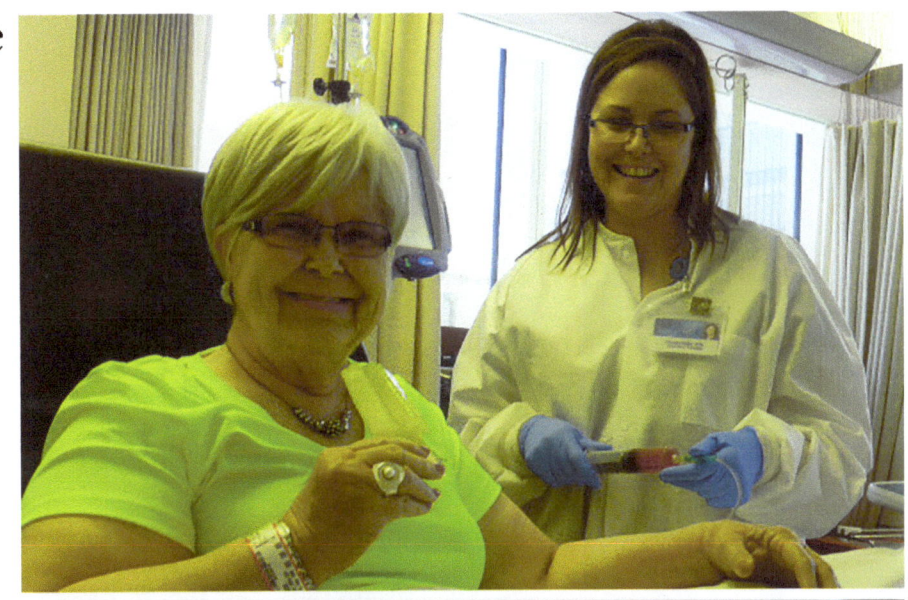

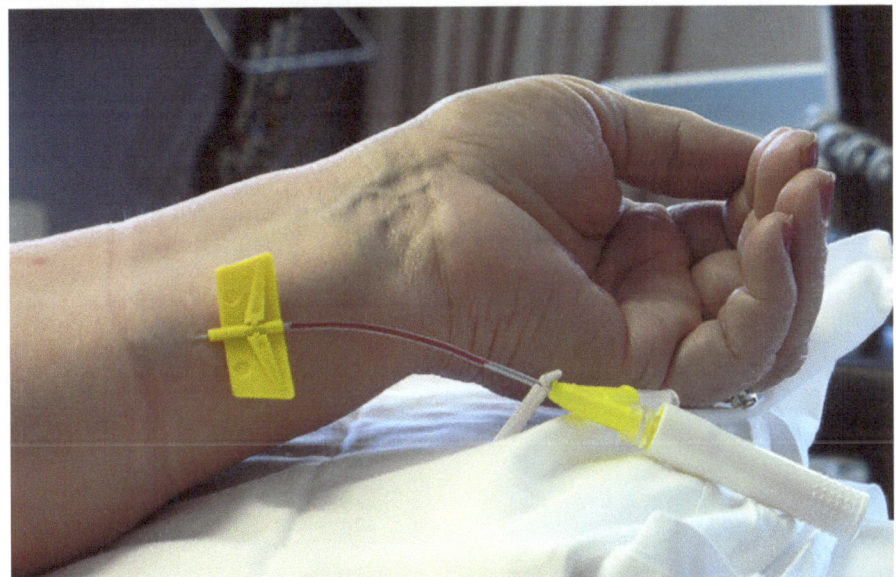

Second E.C. (Epirubicin Cyclophosphamide) Chemotherapy Treatment. | May 5, 2014
Neulasta Booster Shot | May 6, 2014

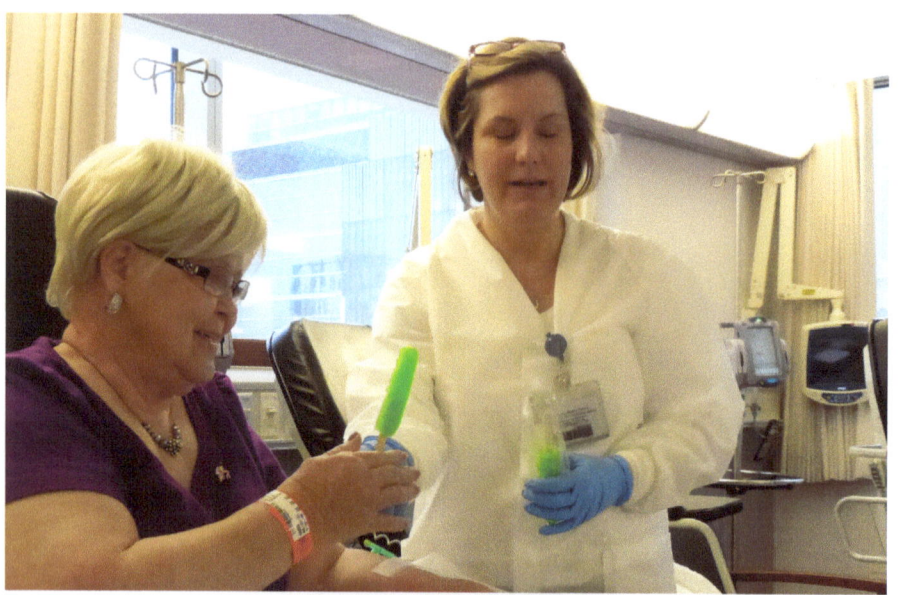

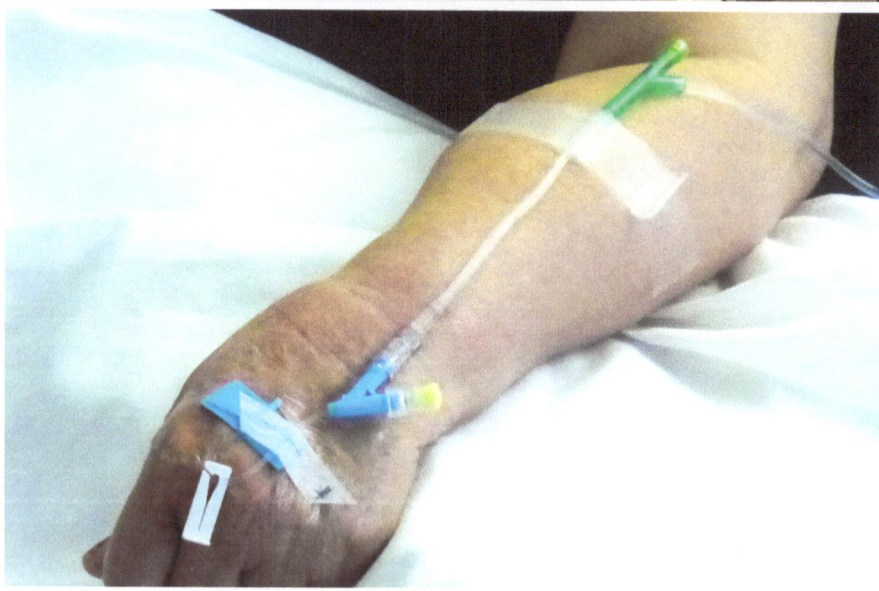

Sacrifices Well Worth Making

While patients travel to the Mayo Clinic from around the world, the cost of doctoring at the Mayo Clinic is really no different than the cost of doctoring anywhere else in the United States. To save money, we would pack sandwiches, skip staying in hotels/motels as much as possible by driving fourteen hours round-trip in a single day, etc. The individualized care that you receive at the Mayo Clinic to combat serious conditions make the sacrifices worthwhile.

Third E.C. (Epirubicin Cyclophosphamide) Chemotherapy Treatment. | May 19, 2014
Neulasta Booster Shot | May 20, 2014

From Chemotherapy
To Radiation

When I was examined at the Mayo Clinic, there was a speck of cancer in one of my lymph nodes. They said that they would wait until after my chemotherapy was complete and do an ultra-sound to see if the treatment had taken care of it. If cancer was still present, they were going to do a double-mastectomy and remove 50 - 60 lymph nodes under each arm.

After completing my chemotherapy treatments, I had an ultra-sound. I was cancer-free. They told me the reason for radiation is to wash away and cleanse all of the chemotherapy out. Sounded good to me, so I proceeded to have thirty radiation treatments.

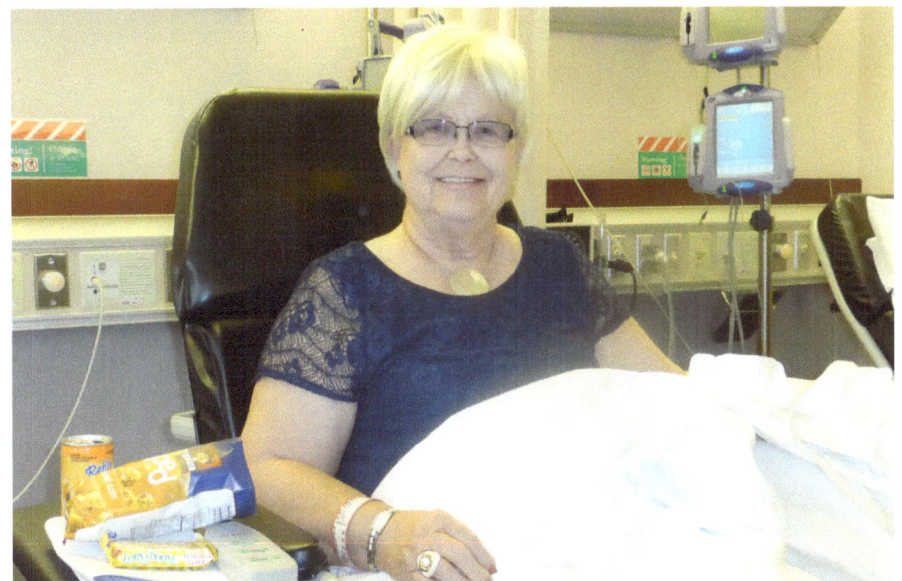

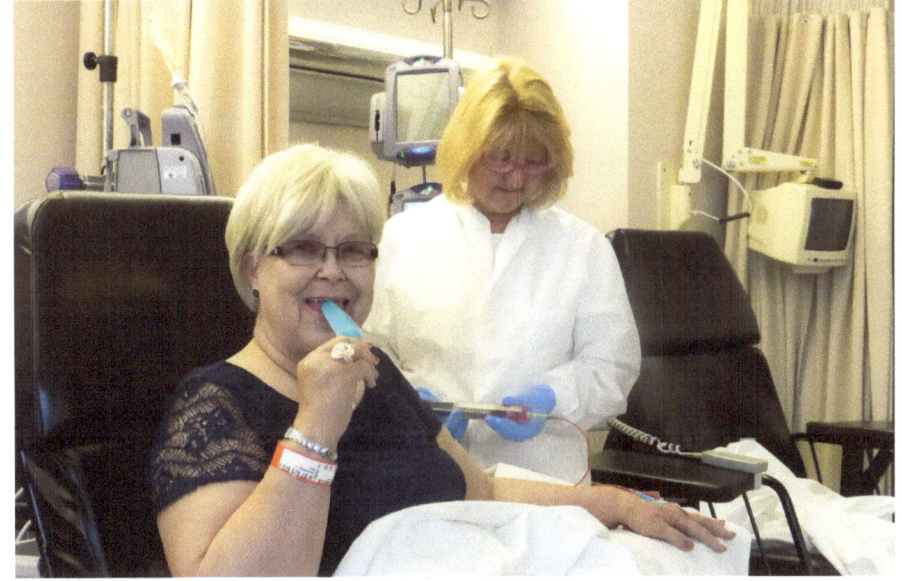

Fourth E.C. (Epirubicin Cyclophosphamide) Chemotherapy Treatment. | June 2, 2014
Neulasta Booster Shot | June 3, 2014

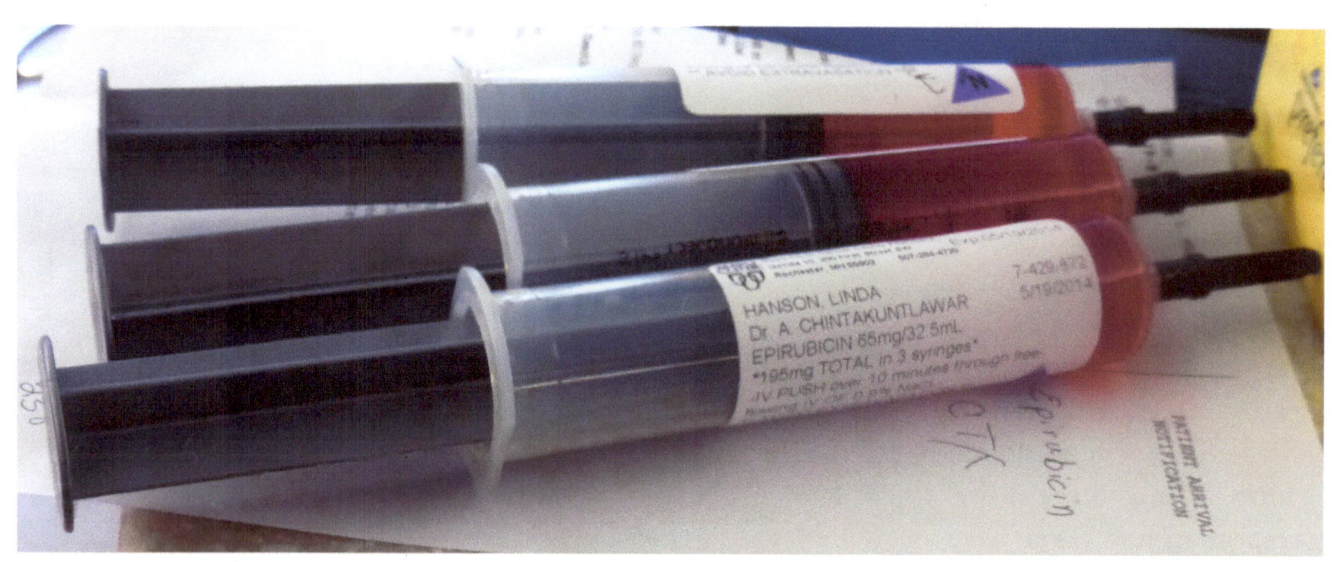

Three syringes injected by a nurse for each Epirubicin Chemotherapy Treatment.

Each I.V., "Push over 10 minutes through free-flowing IV of 0.9% NaCL."

Sucking on popsicles during injections to prevent mouth sores from forming.

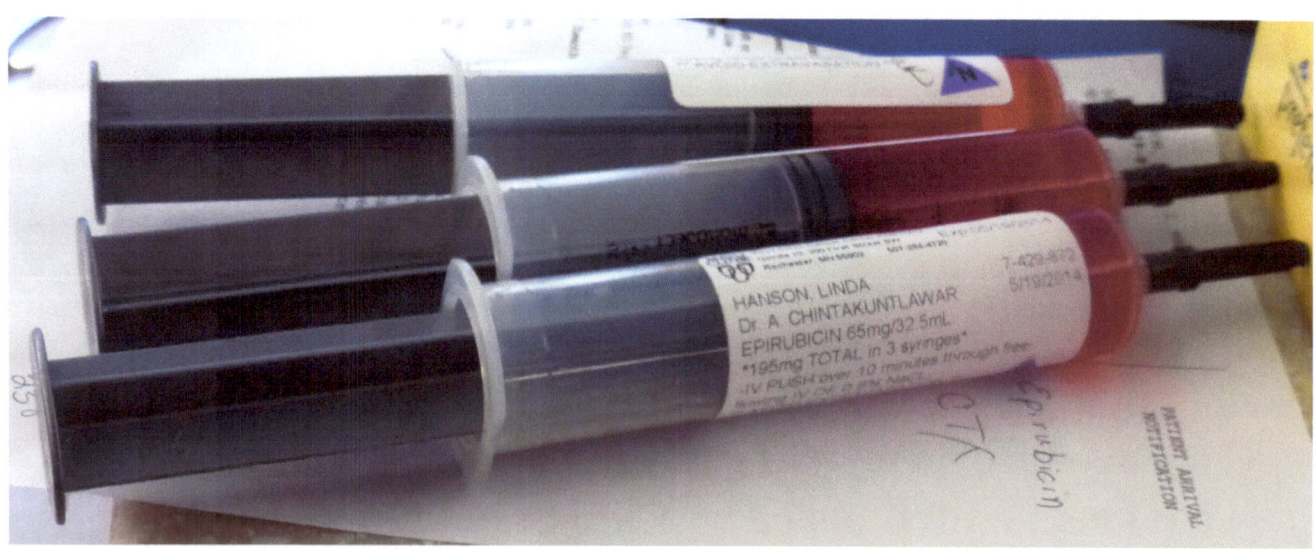

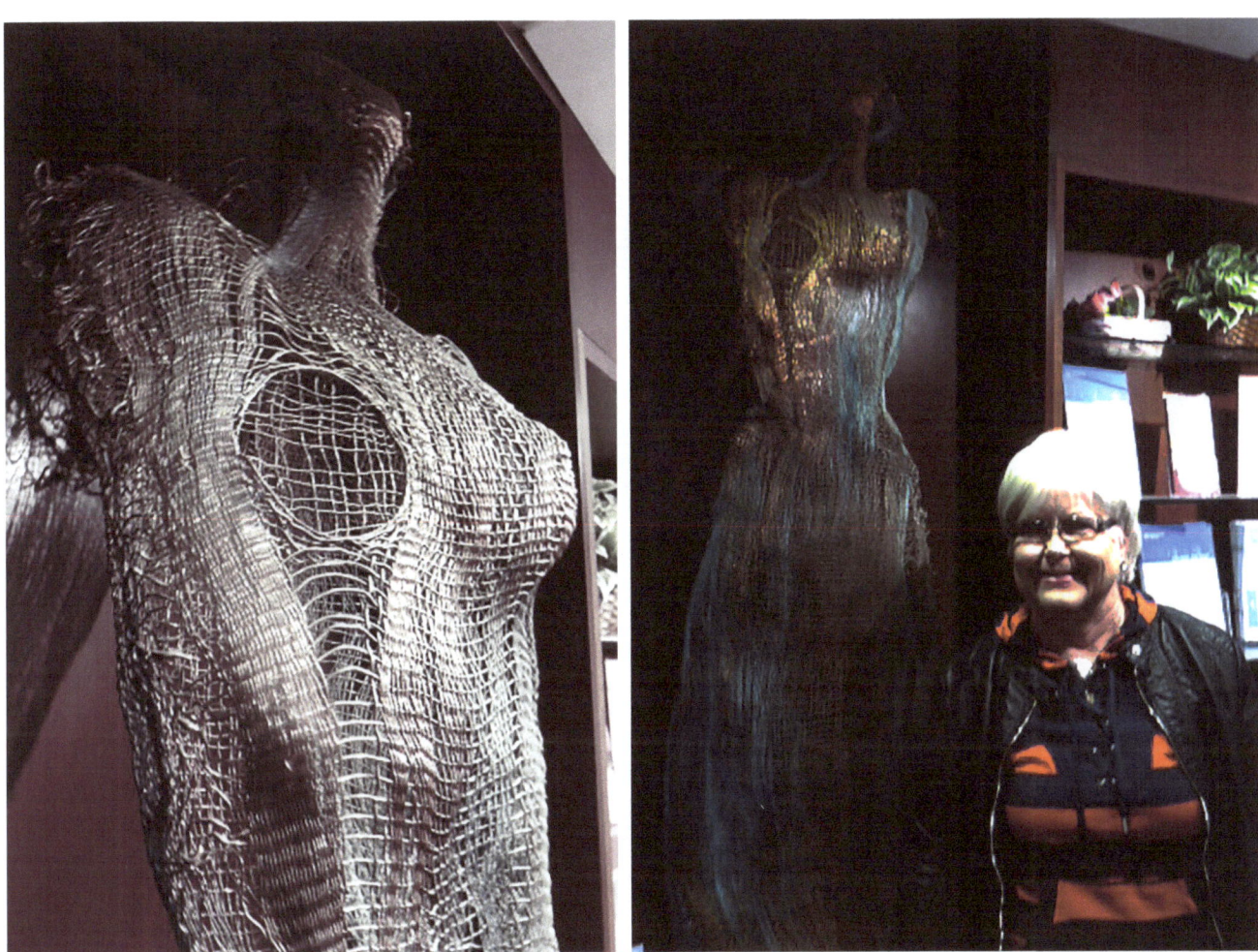

Breast Cancer Statue
Transcendence by Dawn Macnutt of Halifax, Nova Scotia, Canada
Mayo Clinic Cancer Education Center

"This piece was one of twenty-four works of art commissioned for an exhibit entitled Survivors In Search of a Voice. Canadian women artists were asked to create works of art that would give a voice to the thousands of women who had breast cancer. The artists asked breast cancer survivors to "educate" them about their experiences subsequent to being diagnosed with breast cancer."

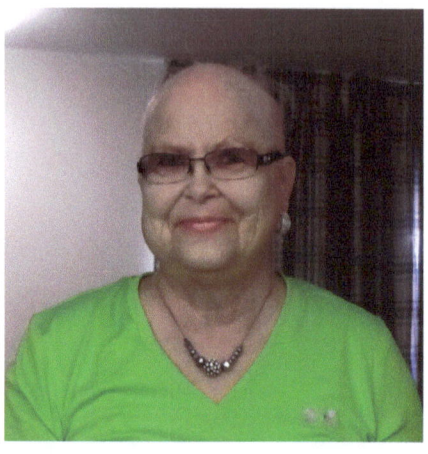
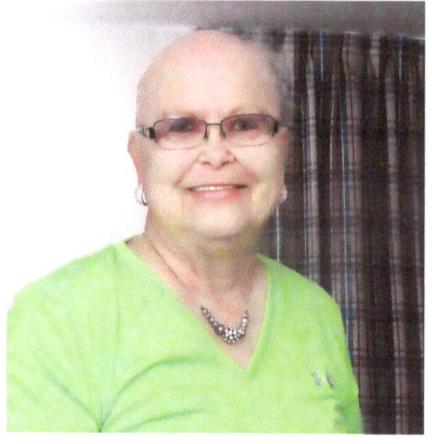
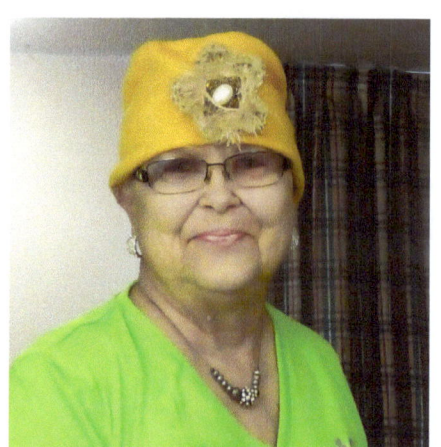

Daily Routine

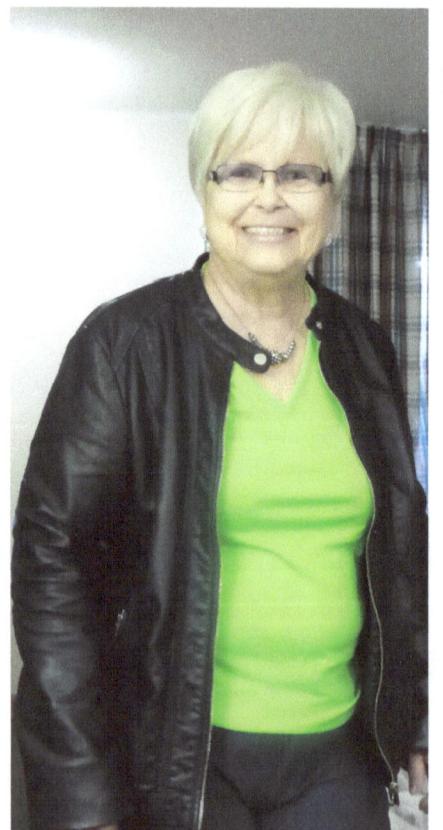

I was told to get white vinegar, dilute it with water, soak a wash cloth in it, lay the wash cloth on my burn for a 15 - 20 minutes a few times a day. It took care of it and healed right away. I noticed several months after radiation, my arms, chest, and back got a dark brown color, almost like a bad sunburn. I could peel that off. It was like a film of something on me. I figured out it was radiation coming out of my system. I had to scrub hard to get it off. I did lose my hair, but not until at the end of some of the chemo treatments that I had. After my tenth chemo, I did develop a red rash on my hands and fore-fingers. I just kept putting lotion on them until it disappeared.

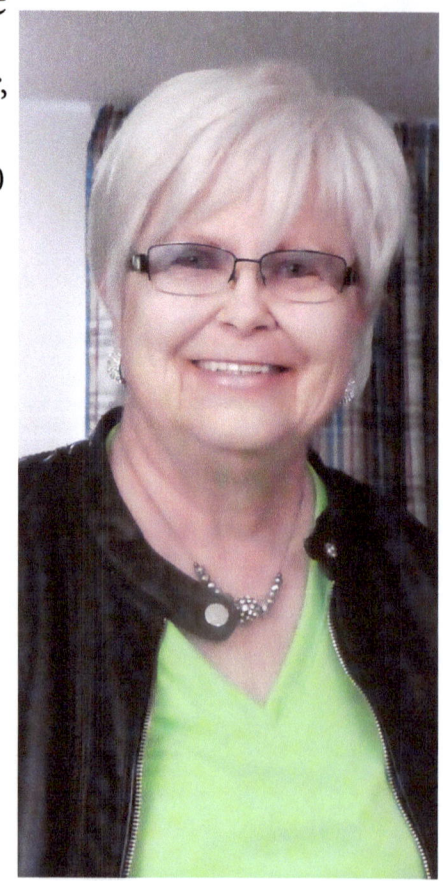

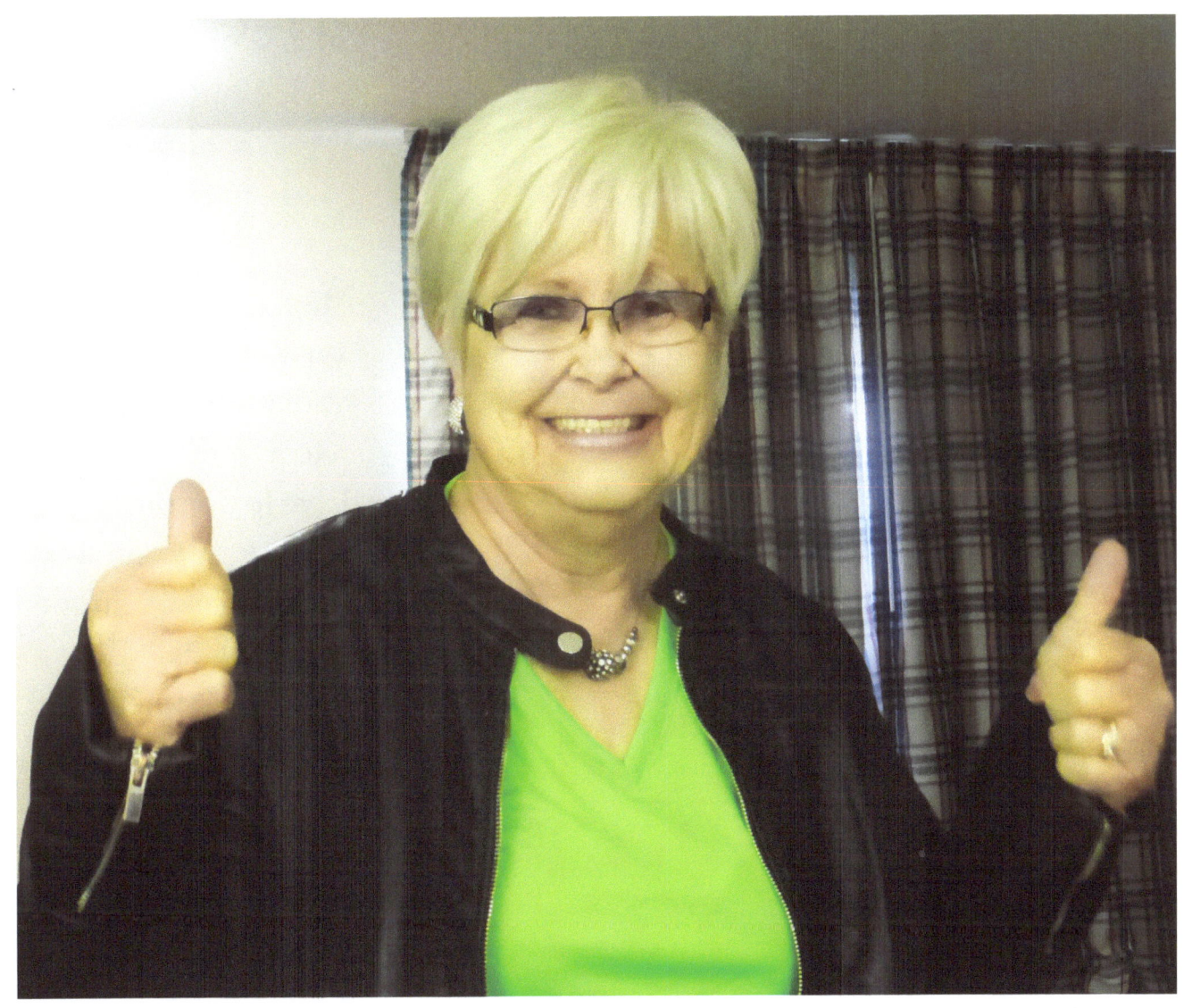

Sixteen Weeks of Chemotherapy Complete!
Clean Bill of Health!
Cancer Free!

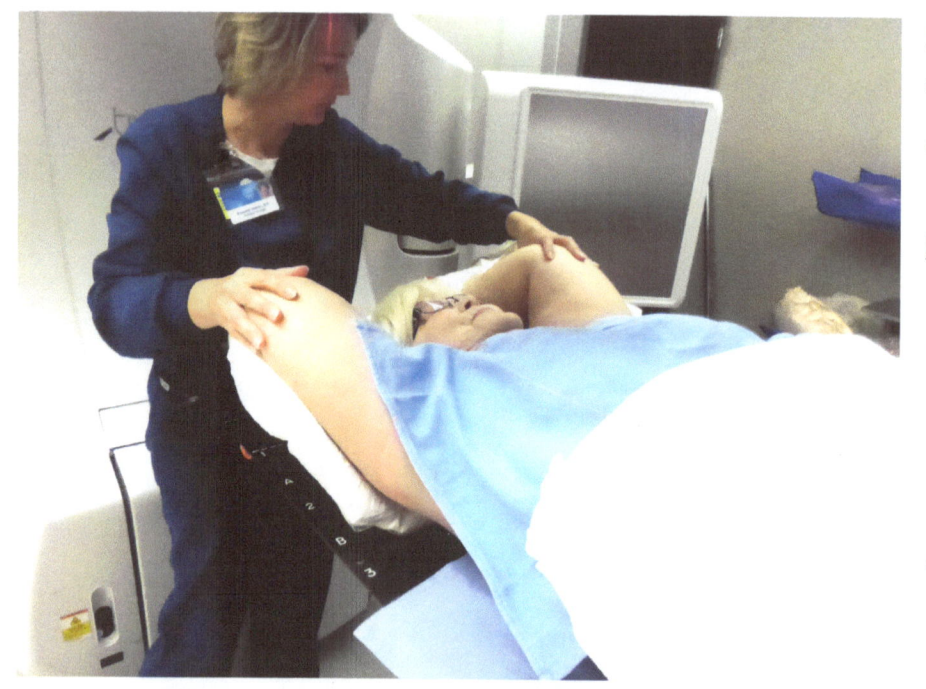

Six Weeks of Thirty Radiation Treatments

June 23, 2014 - August 4, 2014

After a treatment, keep busy. Especially with radiation, I would go to a movie or for a drive to do some sight-seeing. My son was with to chauffeur me around and take me to my appointments. It is important to have a family member or someone with to your appointments to hear what the doctor is telling you, so you don't forget, to help keep it all straight, and helpful when that person takes notes.

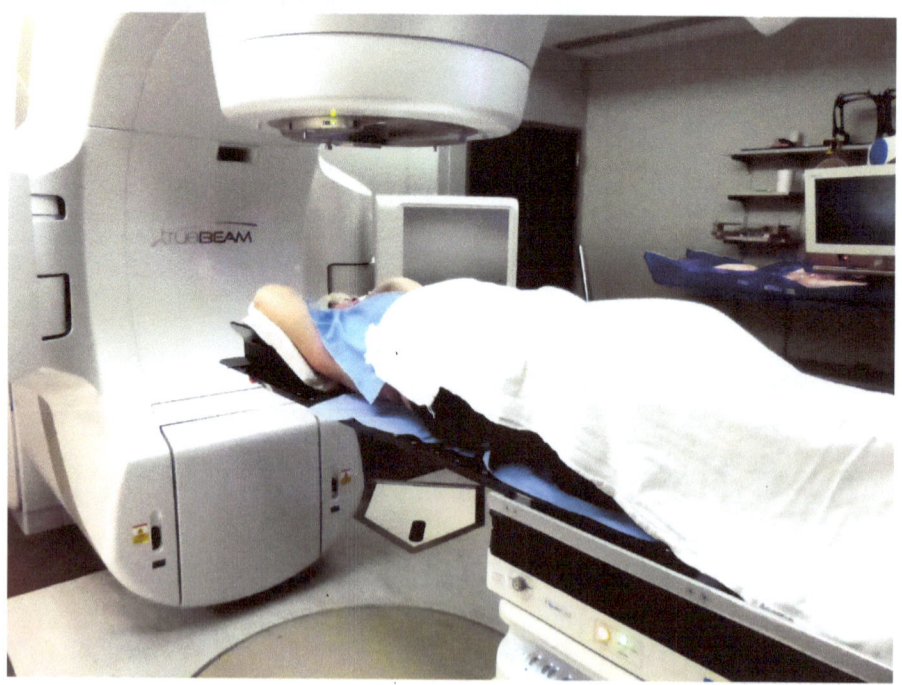

Ring this bell
Three times well
Its toll to clearly say,

My treatment's done
This course is run
And I am on my
way!

— Irve Le Moyne

"The idea for this
celebration was
inspired by Lenny
Rheault, a radiation
oncology patient
and volunteer who
took part in this
tradition when
treated at Mass
General in Boston,
Massachusetts.
This widespread
tradition was
introduced in 1996
at MD Anderson,
Houston, Texas,
when U.S. Navy
Rear Admiral
Irve Le Moyne, a
patient with head
and neck cancer,
installed a brass bell
in the Radiation
Treatment Center."

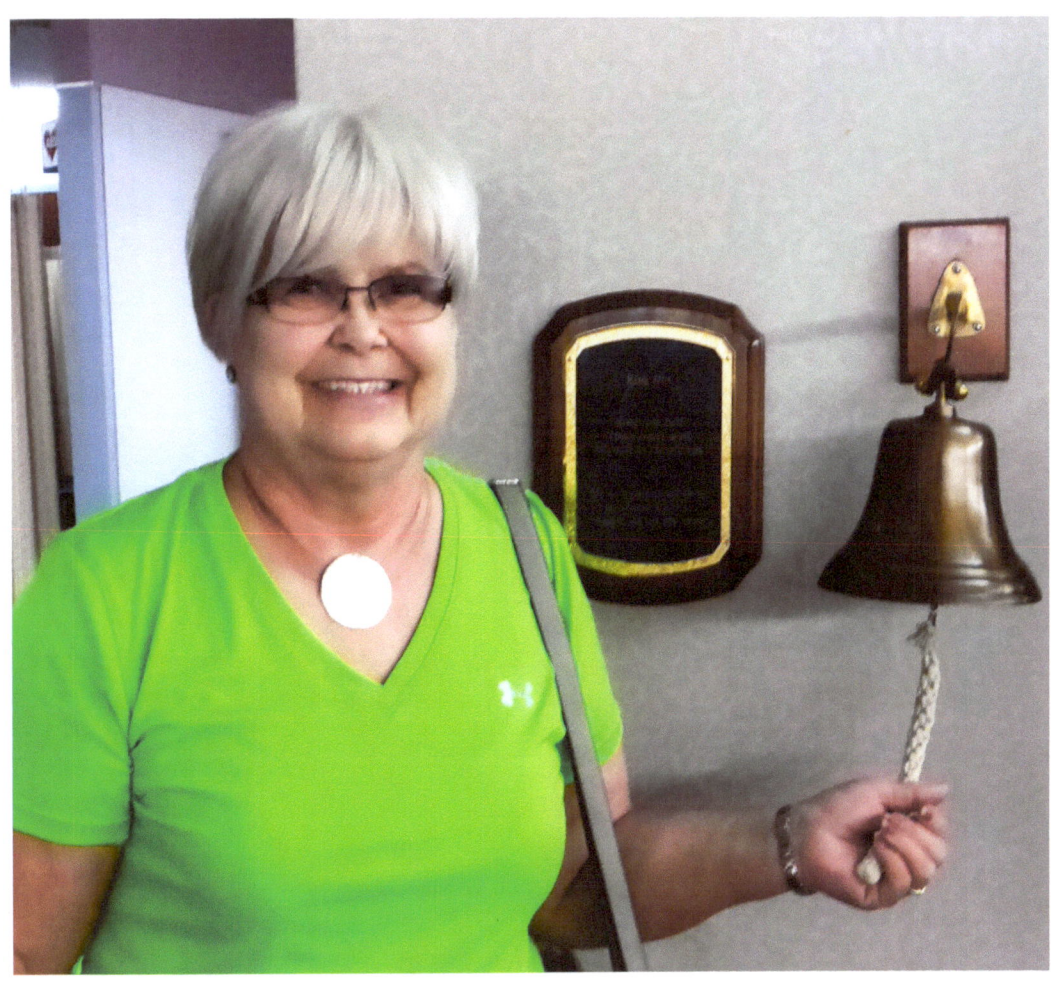

Ringing The Bell
Thirty Radiation Treatments Complete

"The bell is rung three times symbolizing the restoration of balance, harmony and life energy at the end of a patient's radiation treatment."

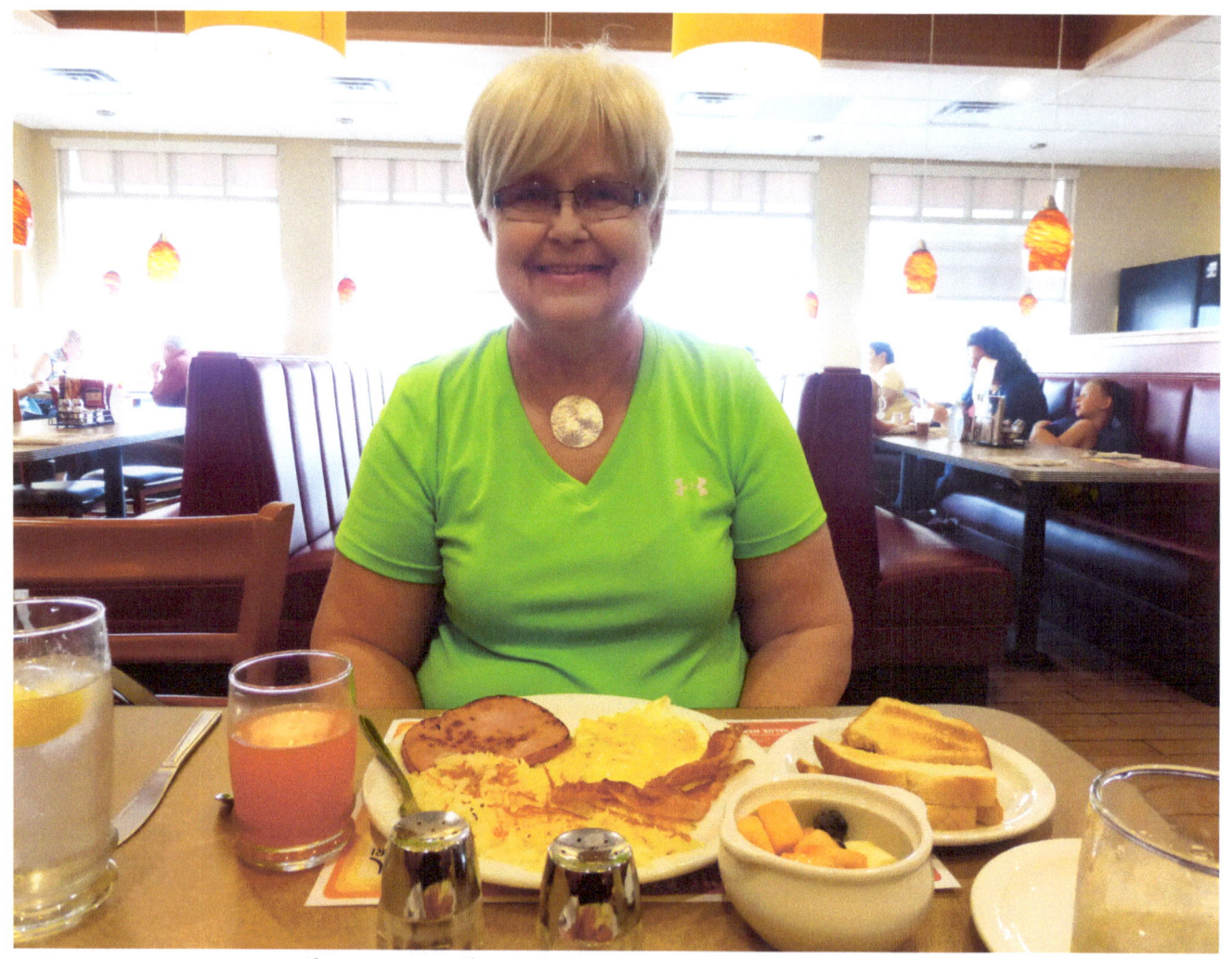

Grand Slam Breakfast

Celebrating The Completion of 16 Chemotherapy & 30 Radiation Treatments.

Ham, Bacon, Sausage, Hash Browns, Eggs, Fruit, Sour Dough Toast, & Grapefruit Juice.

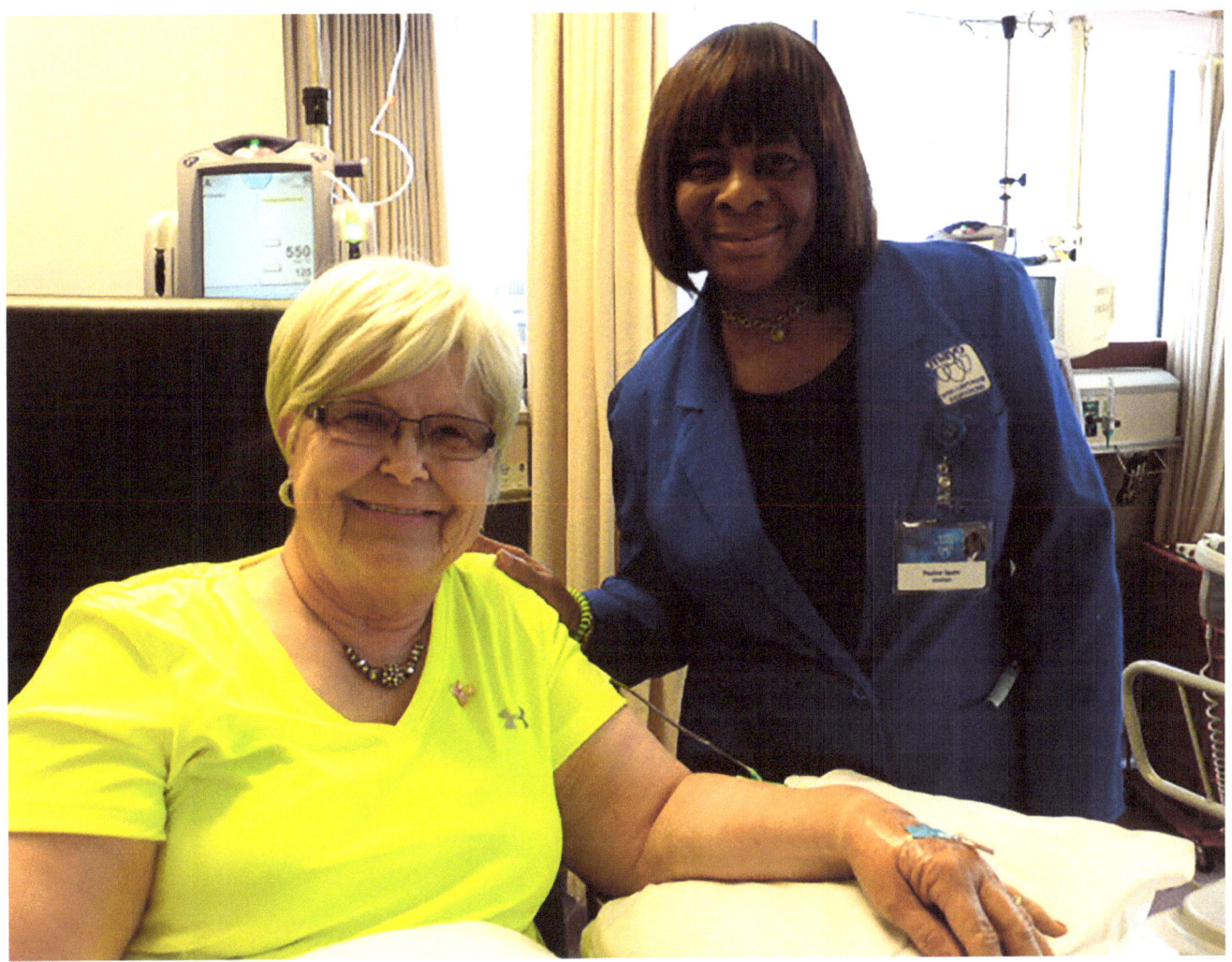

My Favorite Volunteer, Pauline Prince

"Volunteers provide support to patients while they are receiving cancer treatment by offering refreshments, reading material and conversation."

"Mayo Clinic volunteers reassure anxious visitors, provide assistance in expansive surroundings, and offer comfort and amenities during waiting times. They seek to augment the efforts of a caring but busy professional staff to ensure individual attention to the personal needs of Mayo patients."

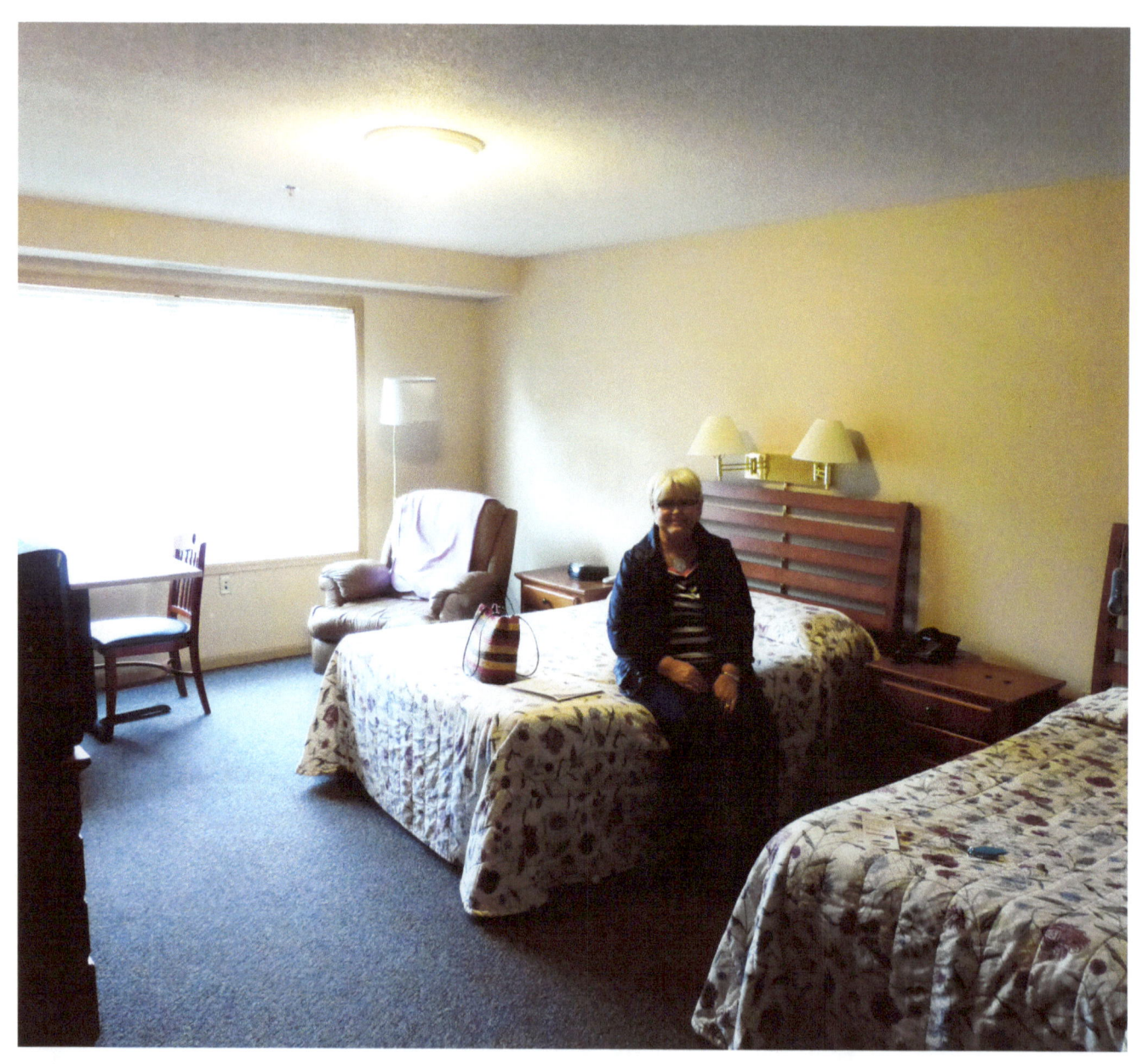

Hope Lodge Room

Sandra J. Schultz Hope Lodge
June 30, 2014 - August 4, 2014

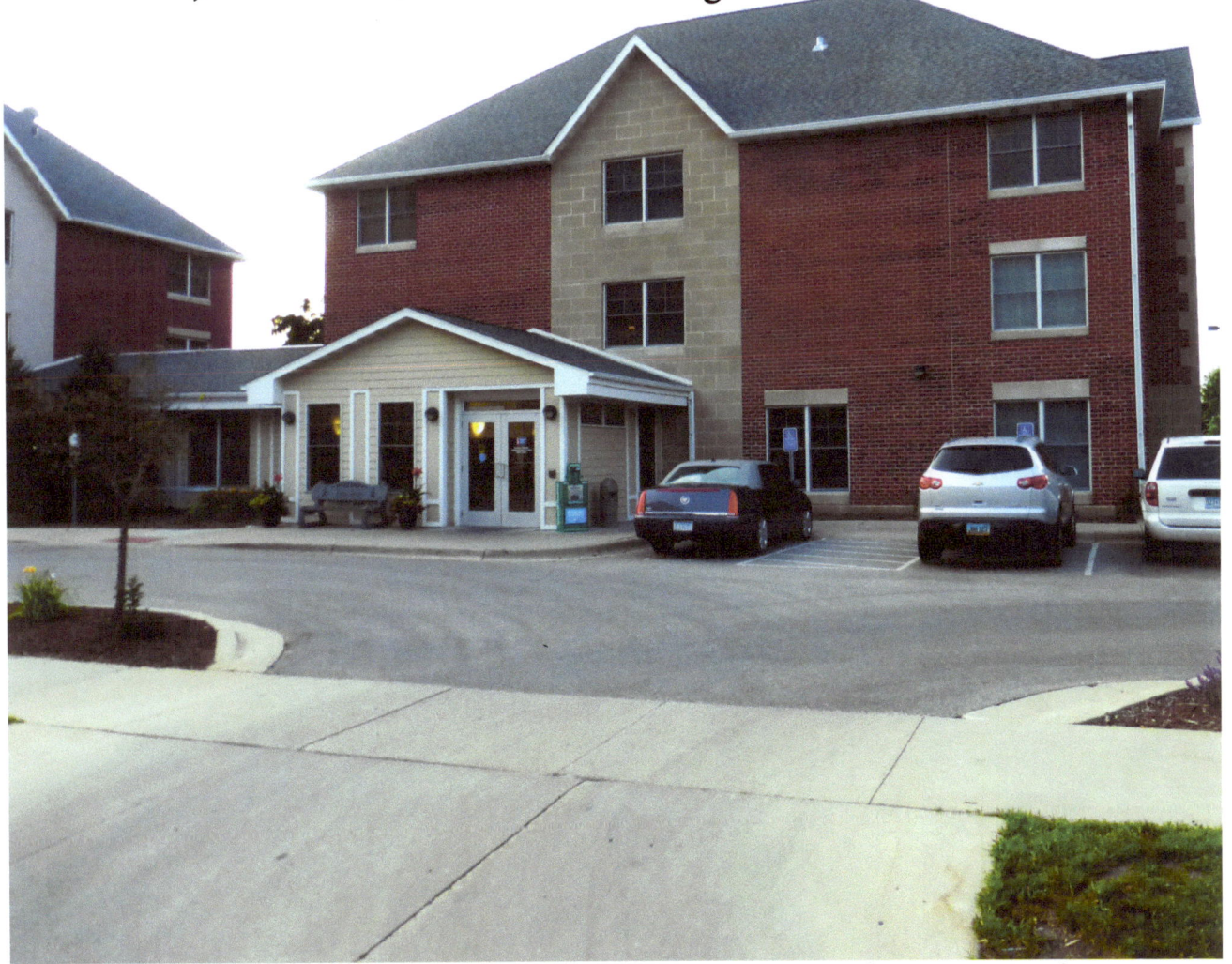

For five of my six weeks of radiation treatments, the Hope Lodge was home. Not sure what we would have done, had it not been for the kindness of a free place to stay extended to us, during this time. What a great place to meet folks who are in the same boat of undergoing radiation treatments.

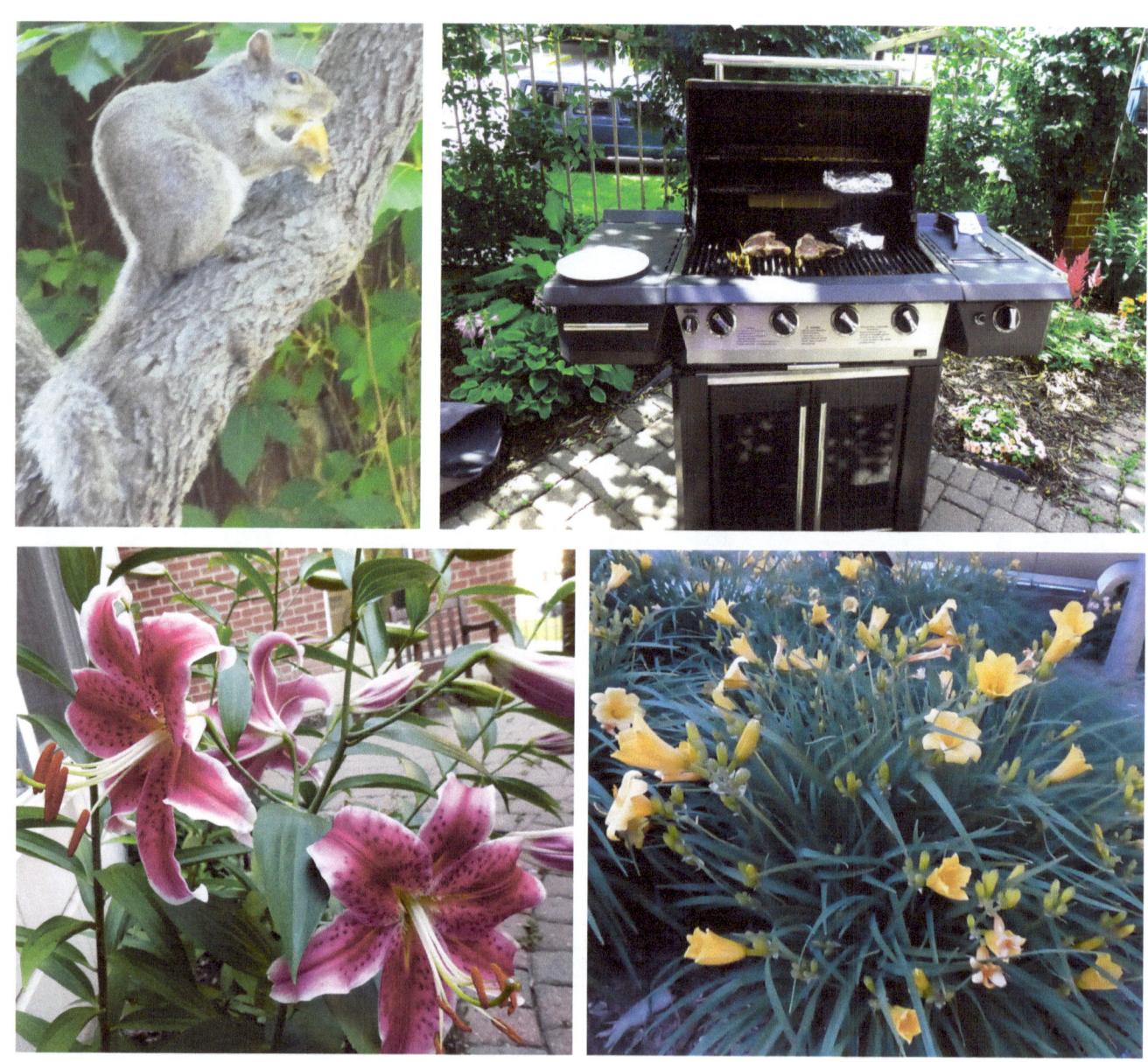

Outside of Hope Lodge

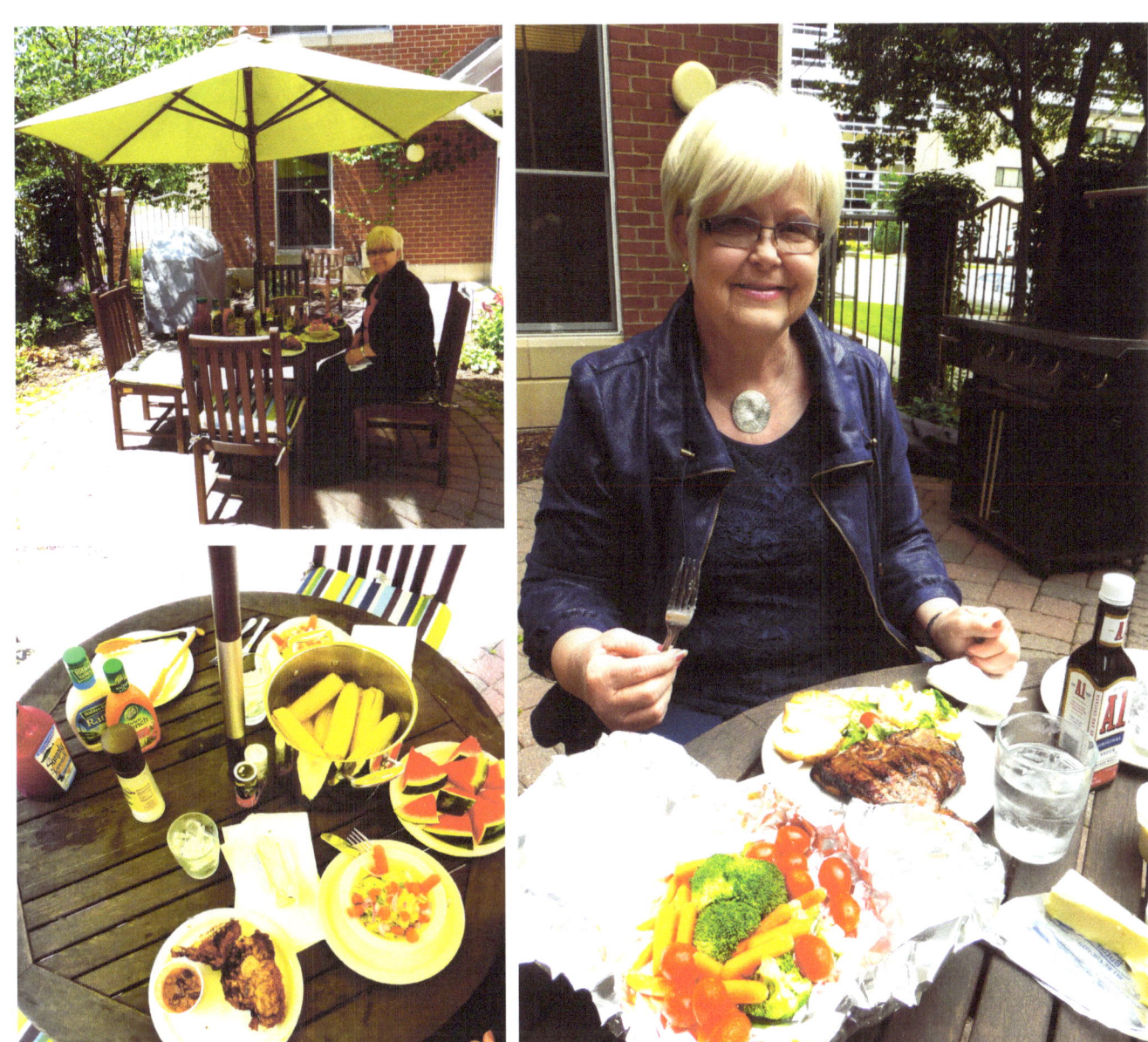

Hope Lodge Outdoor Meals

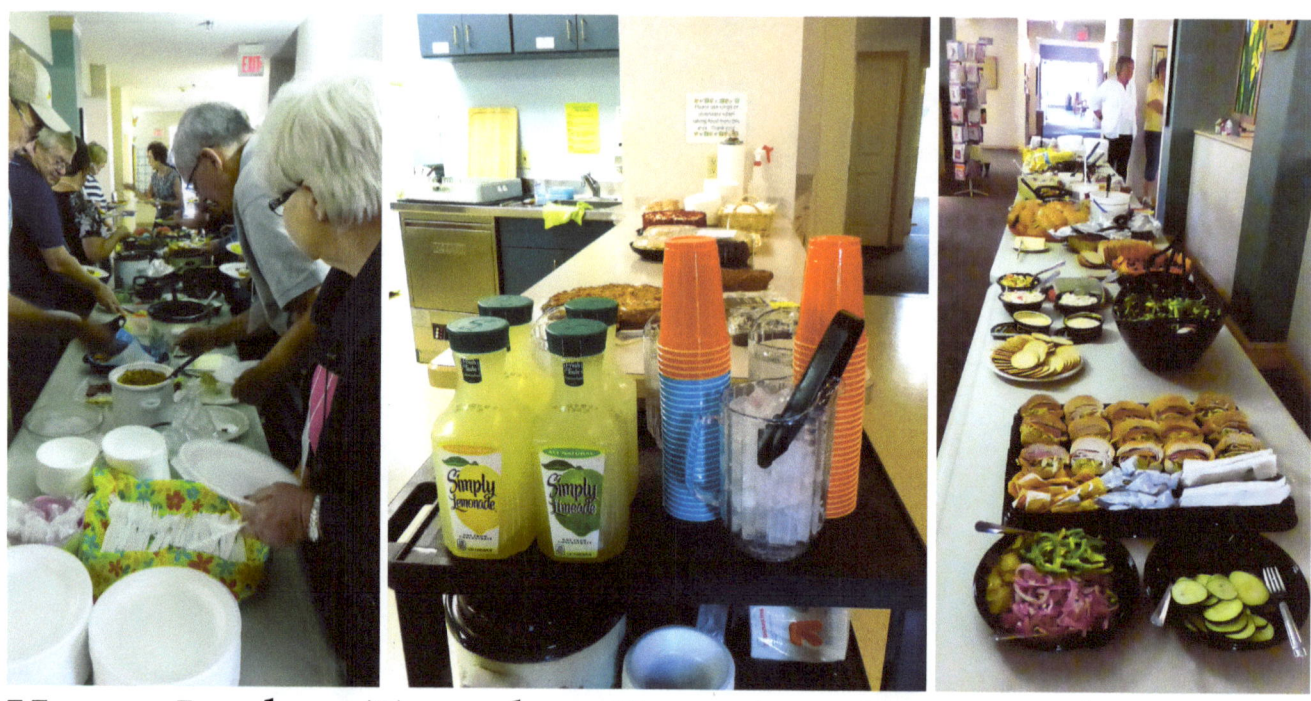

Hope Lodge Tuesday Evening Pot Luck Meals

Tuesday evening pot-luck meals are the best time to get acquainted with other folks, while staying at the Hope Lodge. Beginning at 6:00 p.m., each pot luck meal begins with Hope Lodge volunteers making announcements, asking if it's anyone's last pot-luck meal as a result of their treatments being complete by the following week. If so, the people will share their names, where they are from, and generally speak words of gratitude for staying at the Hope Lodge. Next, Hope Lodge volunteers will ask if it's anyone's first pot-luck. If so, the folks will say who they are, where they are from, and be welcomed with applause.

Everyone lines up for the pot-luck feast. The long tables of food may include: ham, chicken, Subway sandwiches, BBQ's, chips, watermelon, strawberries, vegetable trays, pastas, and pizza. They have a separate area by one of the kitchens for desserts, lemonade, coffee, etc. At about 7:00 p.m., Hope Lodge volunteers will draw names (you register with your name on a slip of paper in a box before eating or before the drawing) for prizes that are donated. These prizes are usually a few nice quilts that have been donated by past Hope Lodge guests or their families or religious groups such as the Mennonites. One week they gave away a diamond necklace from Kay Jewelers, which I was lucky enough to win. The following week, my son won one of the quilts.

Tuesday Evening Entertainment at Hope Lodge

Following the drawings is entertainment at the lodge, ranging from church groups singing beautiful music to a magician. It's a nice evening for all. Occasionally past Hope Lodge guests will donate a catered meal by a local restaurant, such as Victoria's, for folks who are staying at Hope Lodge. Church groups also come in on-occasion to serve meals to Hope Lodge guests.

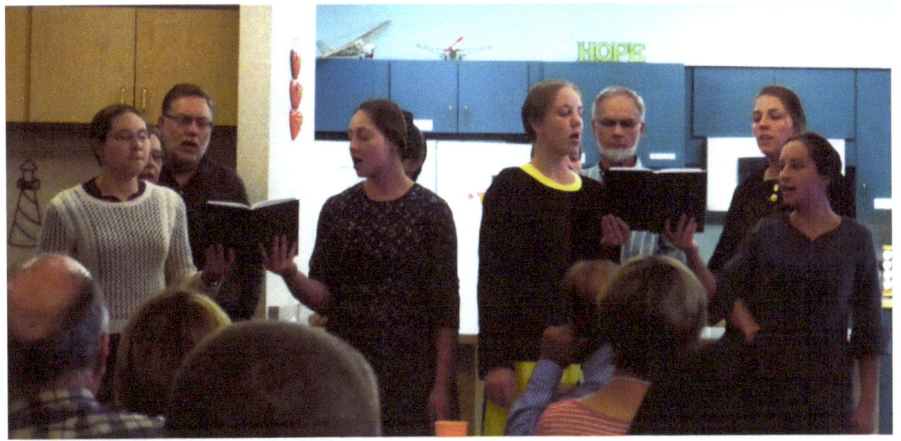

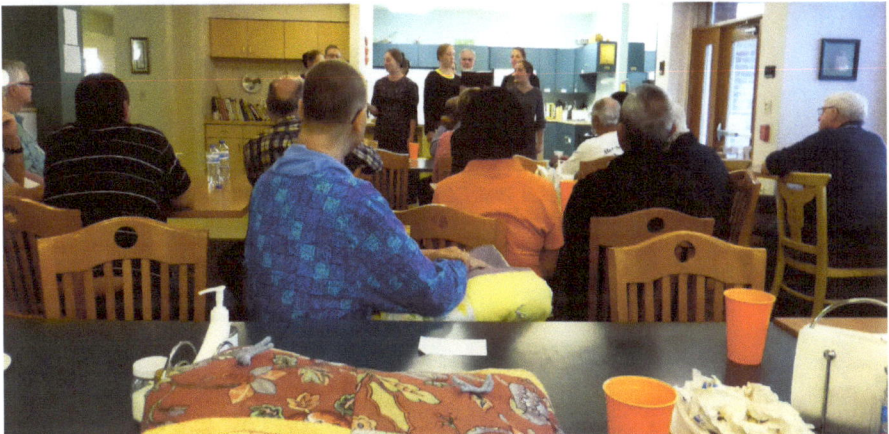

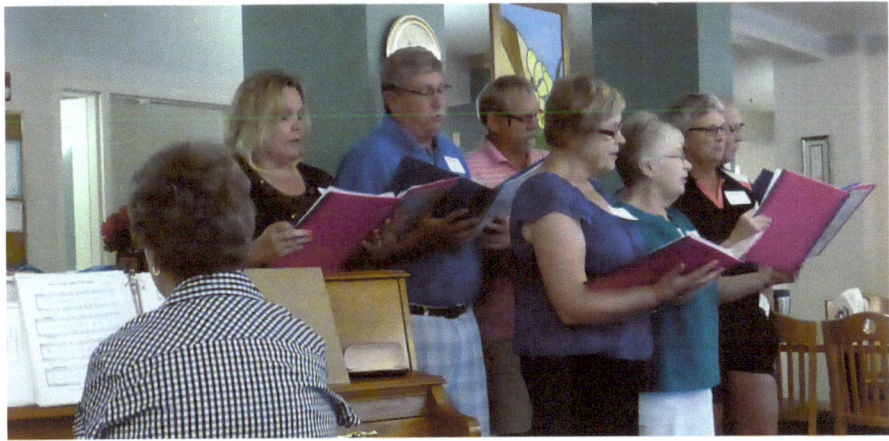

Inside Hope Lodge

Top-Left: Our kitchen area. The Hope Lodge has eight shared kitchens (four pairs), designated by room number. Each room has a designated refrigerator shelf, freezer shelf, and pantry cupboard.

Top-Middle: Looking out at the main indoor dining area from the neighboring kitchen.

Top-Right: Mailboxes. Every week you get a calendar-of-events in your mailbox. The calendar may include free car washes in the parking lot, bible studies, cancer support groups, etc.

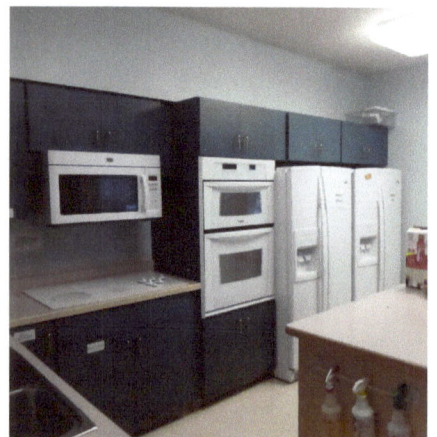 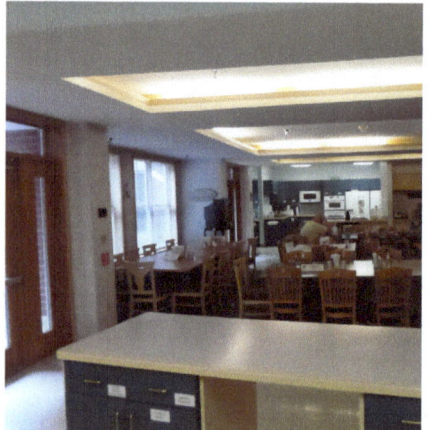 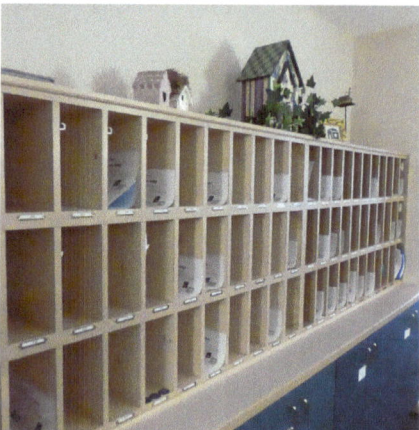

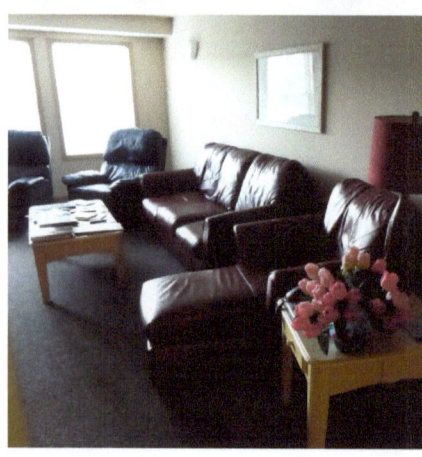 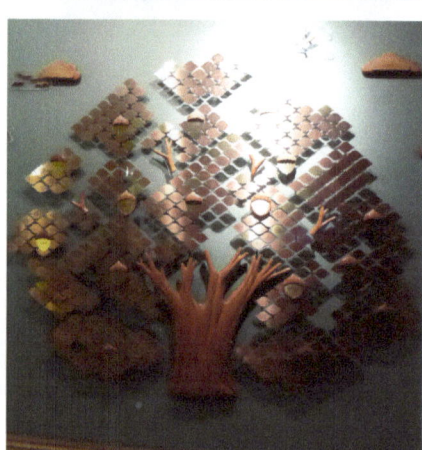 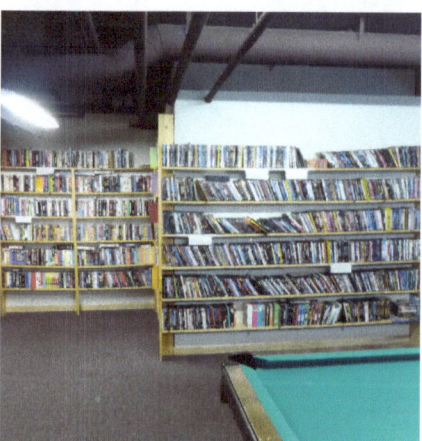

Bottom-Left: Common lounge areas with cable TV on each floor, designed so that Hope Lodge guests will meet and interact with one another. This TV room was on our floor.

Bottom-Middle: One of several beautiful trees with names engraved on each leaf from folks who have made donations to the Hope Lodge.

Bottom-Right: DVD & CD library in the basement for Hope Lodge guests.

"The American Cancer Society Hope Lodge of Rochester, MN, opened its doors in 1999 with 28 rooms available to those patients receiving cancer treatments at the Mayo Clinic. In June of 2007, it was renamed the Sandra J. Schulze American Cancer Society Hope Lodge and was expanded to 60 rooms to meet the growing need of housing for cancer patients and their caregiver. Thanks to their generous support, the family of Sandra J. Schulze made the expansion of the building possible."

Sandra J. Schulze Hope Lodge

"Sandra was a woman you would never forget once you met her. She was Sandy to everyone and she never forgot a face. Her warm smile, compassionate manner, wise eyes and gentle touch always let you know she was listening and interested in you. She made you feel special.

The Sandra J. Schulze Hope Lodge, a concept of the American Cancer Society, is the outcome of the generosity of the citizens of Rochester, the compassion shown by the Mayo Foundation and the Schulze family. It is a true partnership of caring and a perfect reflection of Sandy's special way of helping others cope with the treatments needed to battle this difficult disease.

Sandy was born in Hopkins, Minnesota on December 11th, 1940 and lived most of her life in Minnesota. She earned her Associates Degree from the University of Minnesota and married Richard Schulze on June 2nd, 1962. Sandy had four children and five grandchildren when she passed away on June 21st, 2001 of Mesothelioma, a cancer caused by asbestos.

Sandy's life was exciting and busy! She stayed at home with her children and while raising them she supported, encouraged and assisted her husband with his career in building Best Buy Co., Inc. She loved to visit the stores and talk with store employees and their families, she considered them a part of her family.

Sandy cared deeply about others and was always quick to offer a helping hand and words of encouragement along with a friendly smile. She was truly touched by the many people she knew who were affected by cancer. Trying her best to add support and cheer to their lives she cared for them with visits, phone calls, letters of hope and with prayers. When she was diagnosed with cancer in December of 2000 her six month battle was short but reminded us all to live each day to its fullest.

Mayo Clinic was valiant in their effort to save Sandy. The Schulze Center of Novel Therapeutics was a gift to Mayo by her family in the belief that some cancers will be cured and that Mayo's talented scientists and physicians will find a way.

Sandy's wish for you would be that you find strength, encouragement, compassion, camaraderie and faith during your stay at the Hope Lodge. Sandy and her family wish you peace, hope and good health as you leave the doors and continue your journey."

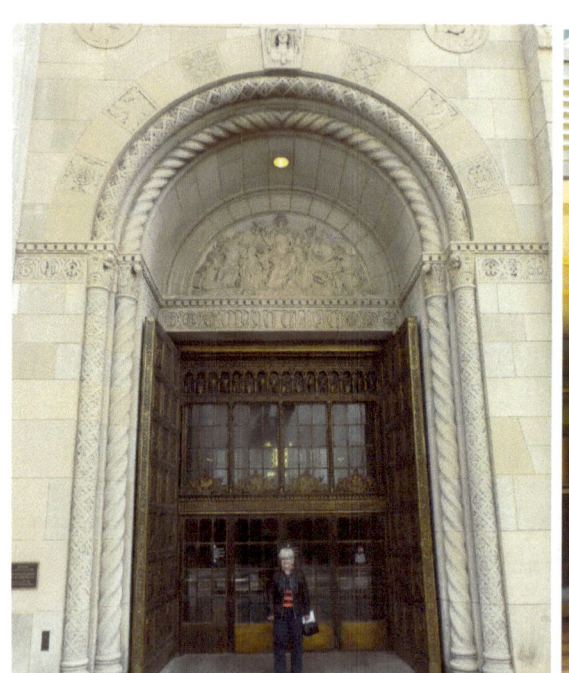
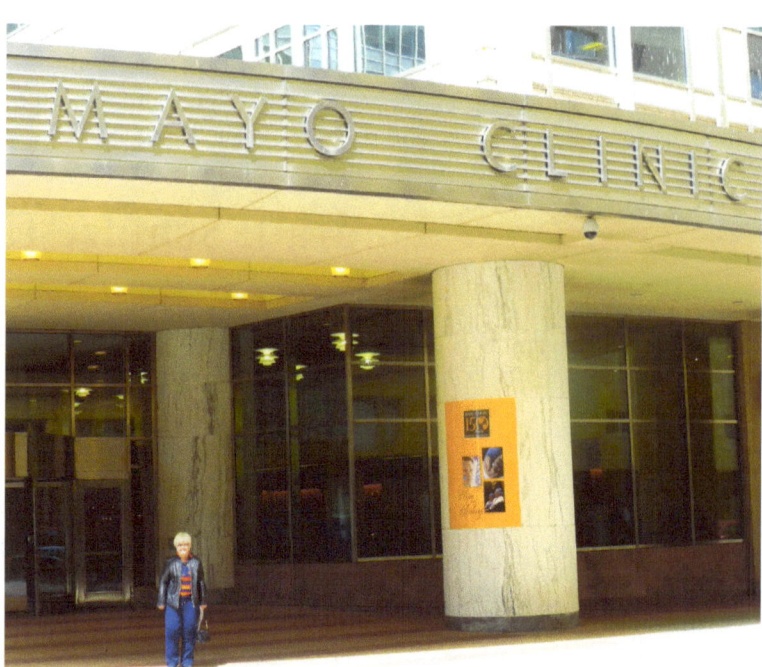
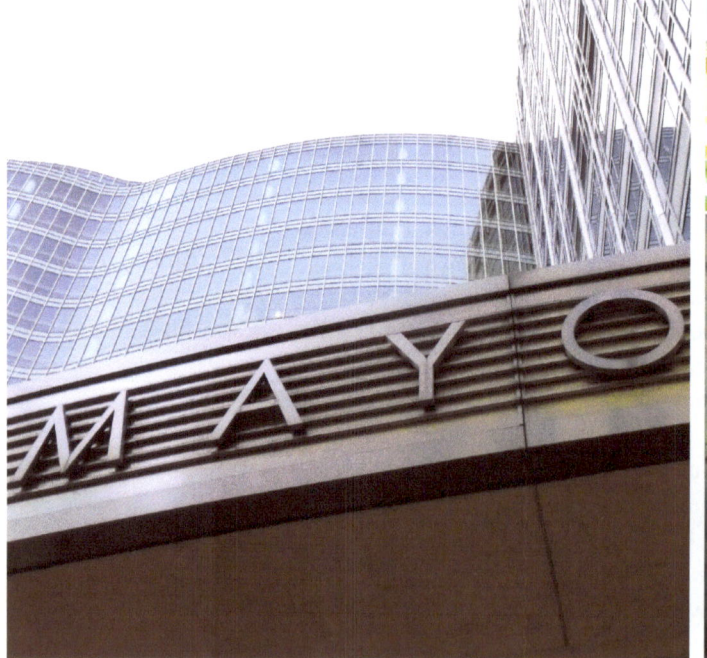
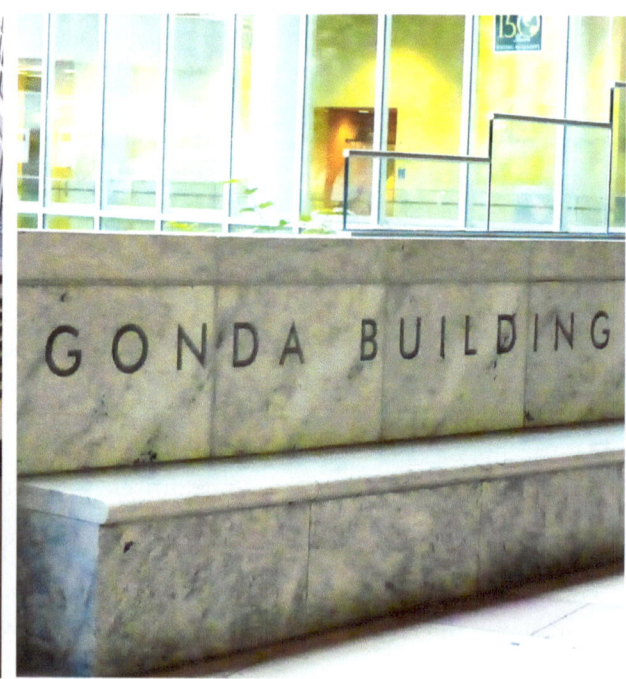

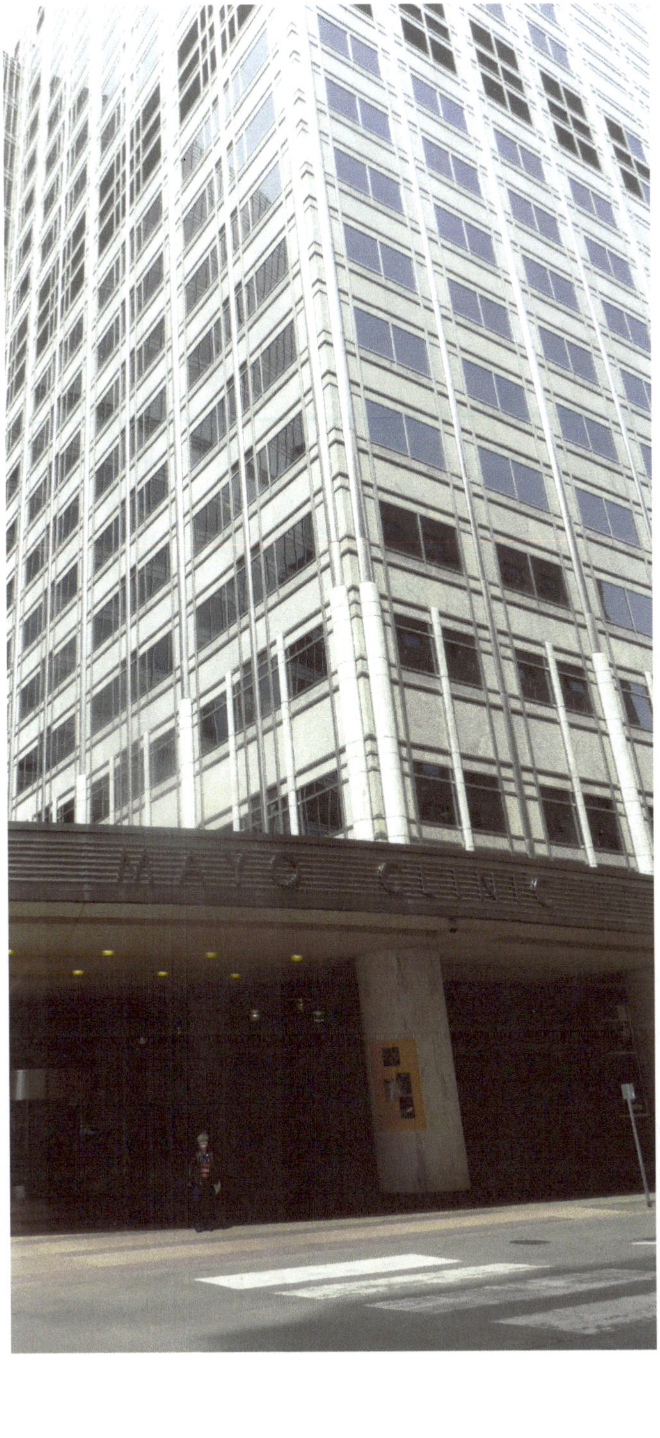

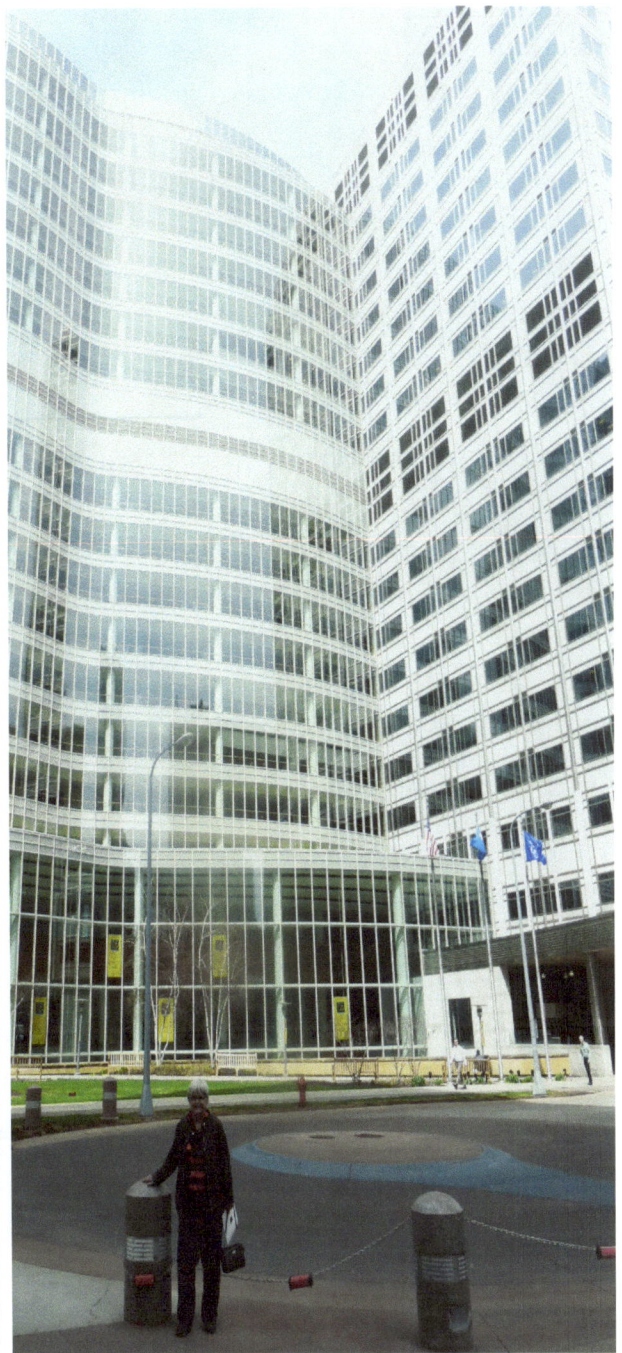

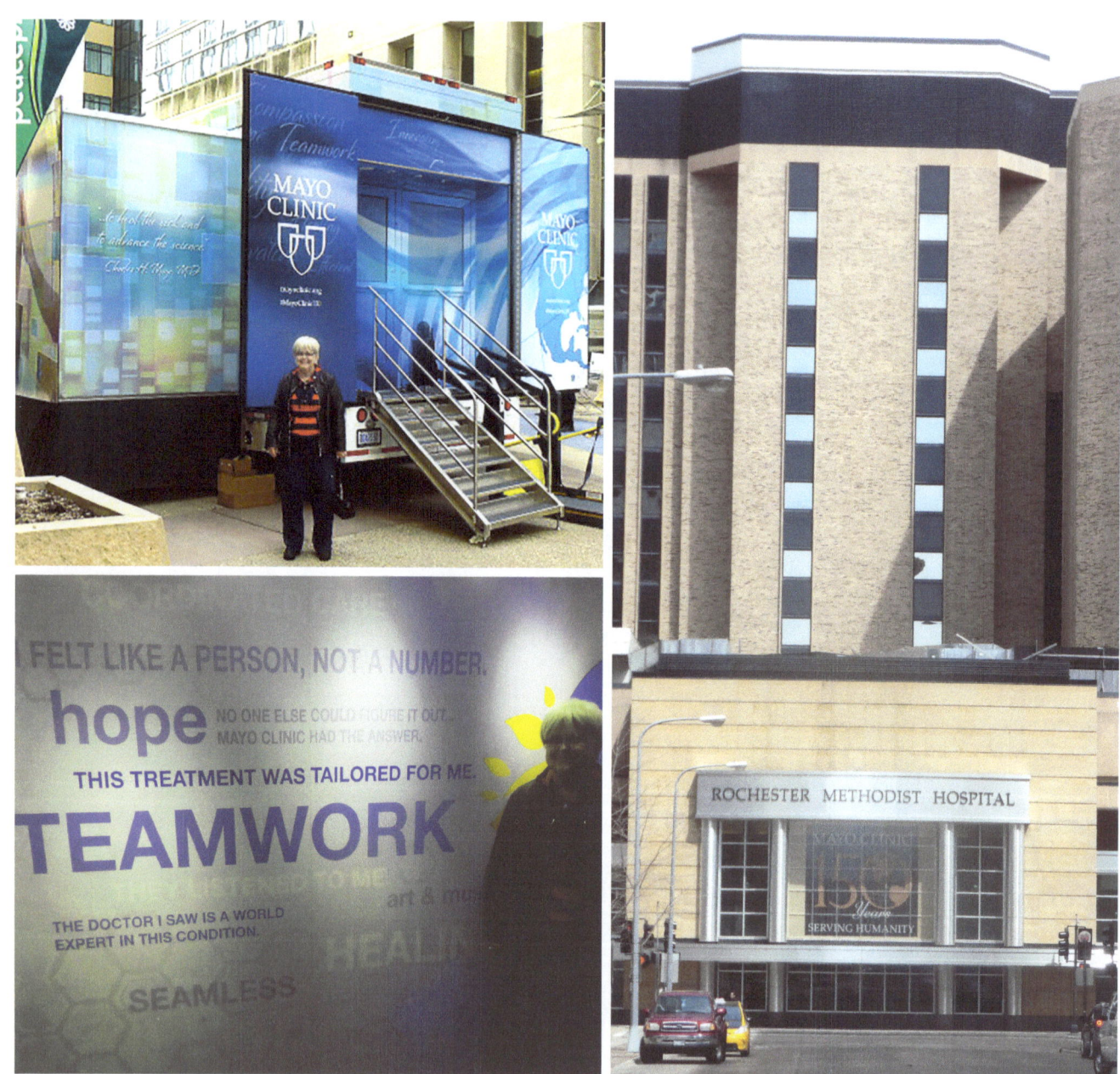

Mayo Traveling Exhibit & Methodist Hospital

Charles (L -born 1865) & William (R - born 1861).

"These brothers from Le Sueur, themselves sons of esteemed doctor and British expat William Worrall Mayo, co-founded the Rochester clinic that bears their namesake, which is now known worldwide for its advances in medical practice and research. It is frequently ranked as one of the best (if not the best) hospitals in the country."

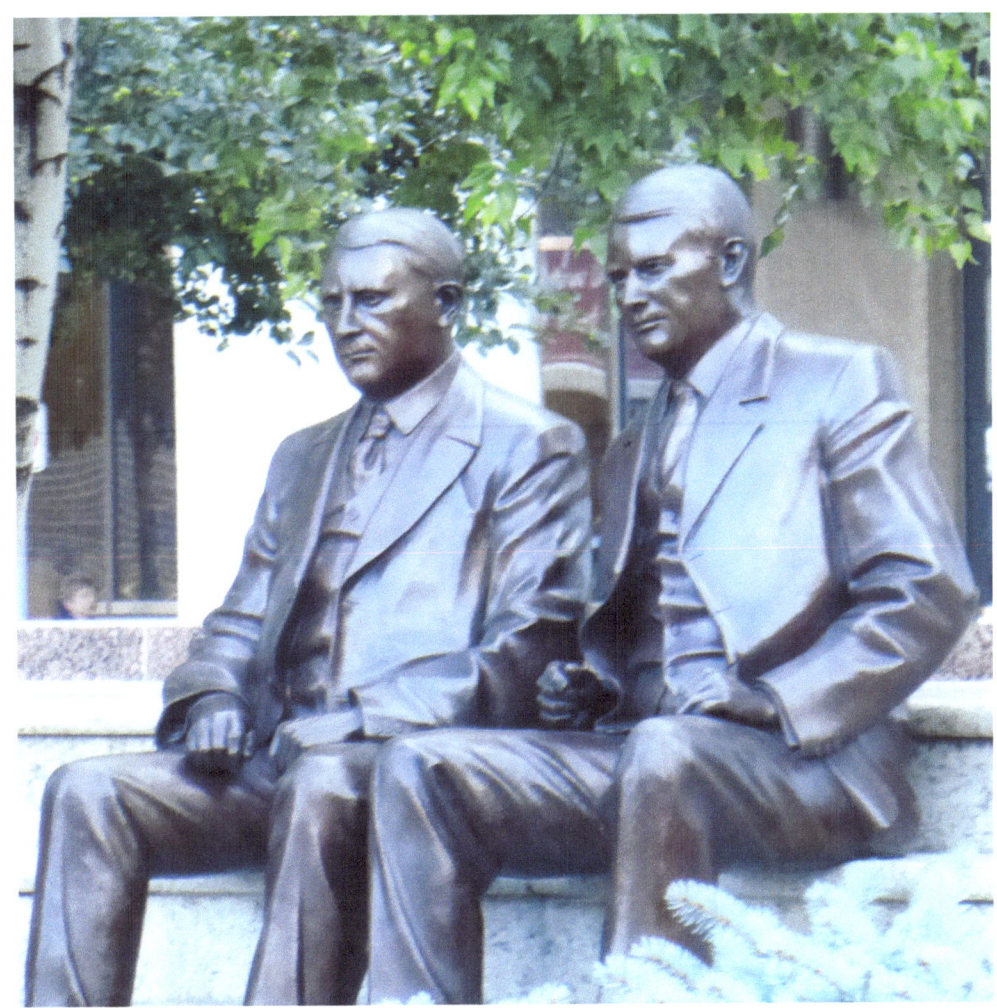

Charles & William Mayo

"On August 21, 1883, a terrible tornado struck Rochester, killing 24 people and seriously injuring over 40 others. One-third of the town was destroyed."

"Doctors William J. Mayo and Charles H. Mayo led the efforts to tend to the victims of the tornado outbreak. It was quickly realized that there were not enough doctors to help the injured, so Mother Alfred Moes and her Sisters of Saint Francis, assisted in giving medical attention to the numerous tornado victims."

"It quickly became evident that a city the size of Rochester needed a hospital. The sisters and doctors got together to form a hospital which later became the world famous Mayo Clinic."

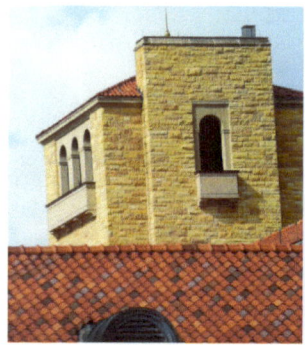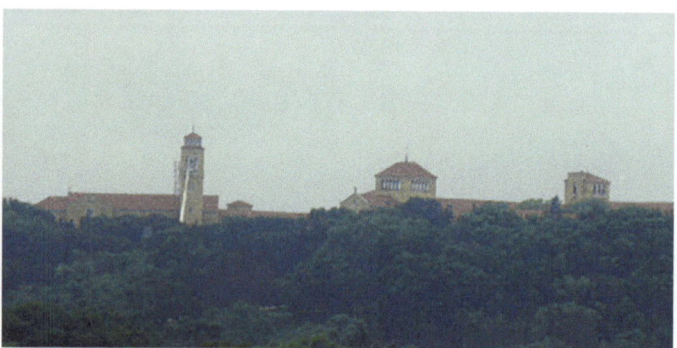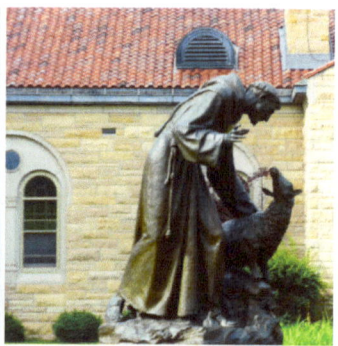

Assisi Heights & Sisters of Saint Francis

- "In 1877, Sister Mary Alfred Moes (shown right), along with her birth sister, Sister Barbara Moes, and 23 other Franciscan Sisters from Joliet, Illinois, came to Rochester, Minnesota, to establish a new community of Franciscan Sisters ready to serve as teachers."
- "In 1883, Rochester was hit by a devastating tornado. The Franciscan Sisters provided care for the victims. Seeing the necessity for health care in the Rochester area, Mother Alfred persisted until Dr. William Worrall Mayo agreed to serve as director of a hospital to be built by the Sisters."
- "Established in 1889, Saint Marys Hospital was on the cutting edge of health care. Today, Saint Marys is part of the Mayo Clinic, serving people from all over the world."
- "The Sisters also continued their work in education, staffing parochial schools in Minnesota and beyond, while also establishing academies in Owatonna and Rochester. Their work included post-secondary education, and in 1894, they founded what would become the College of Saint Teresa in Winona, Minnesota."
- "After the Second Vatican Council (1962-1965), many Sisters entered into areas of social service, spiritual care and went into service abroad. Others continued their ministries in health care and education."
- "The value of the work of the Sisters' teaching cannot be overestimated. The education they provided in these institutions made those they taught ready to pick up the reins and fill the needs of the parishes after Vatican II."
- "The Sisters continue to be involved in the world, partnering with the poor and vulnerable, offering a voice on behalf of those who have none. They are diverse in their personalities and ministries, yet are united by faith in God, the Franciscan tradition, and the heritage of service passed on to them by their Foundress, Mother Alfred Moes."

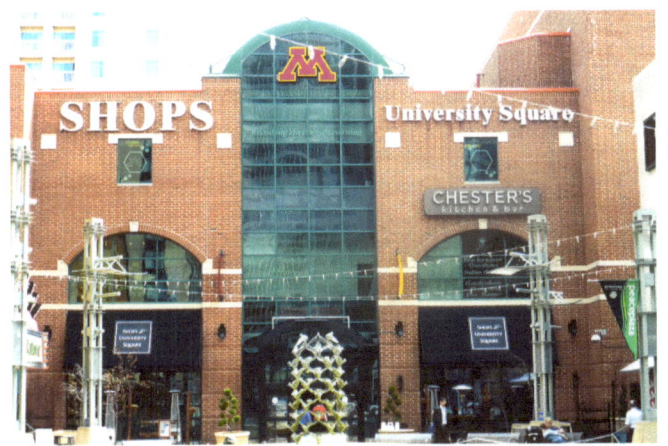

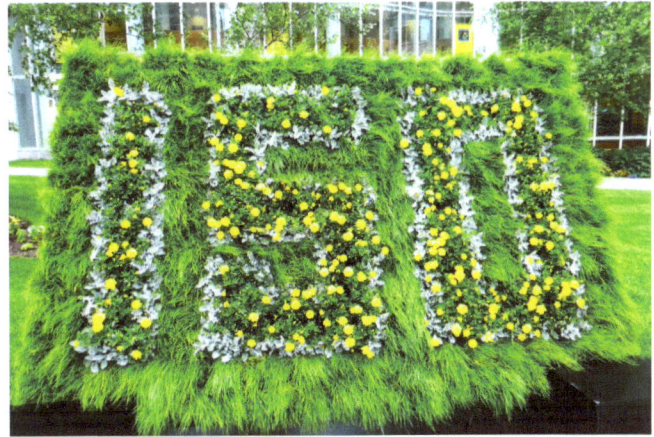

Peace Plaza

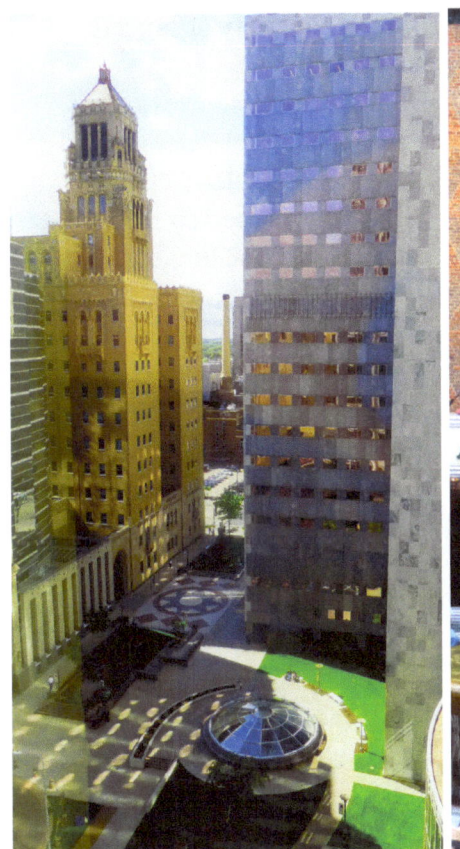

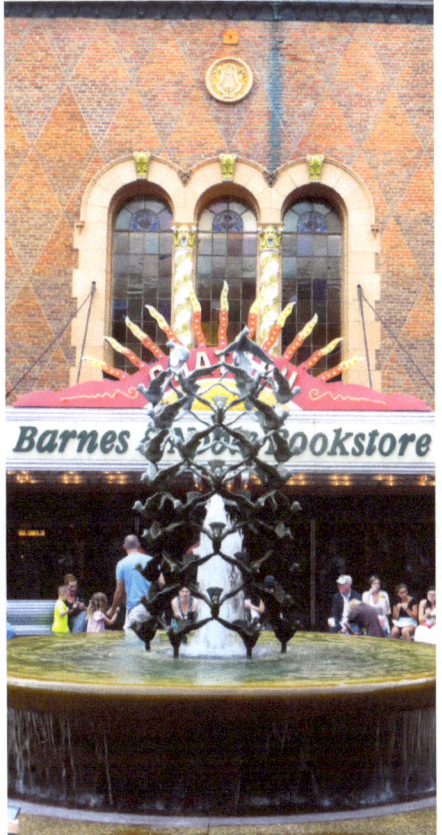

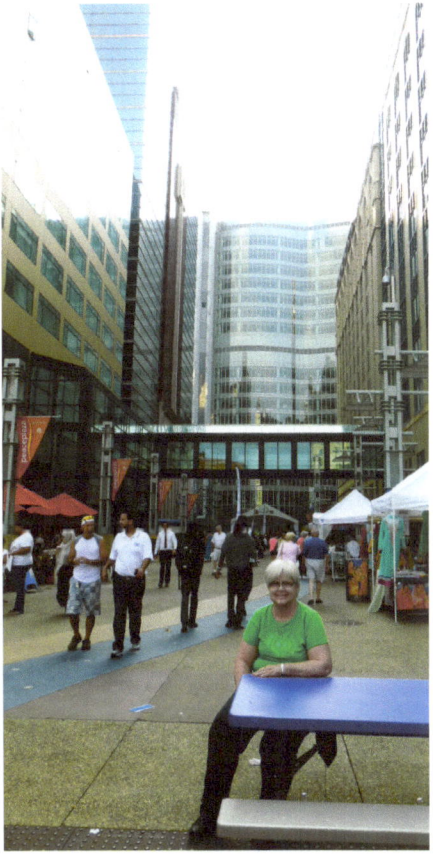

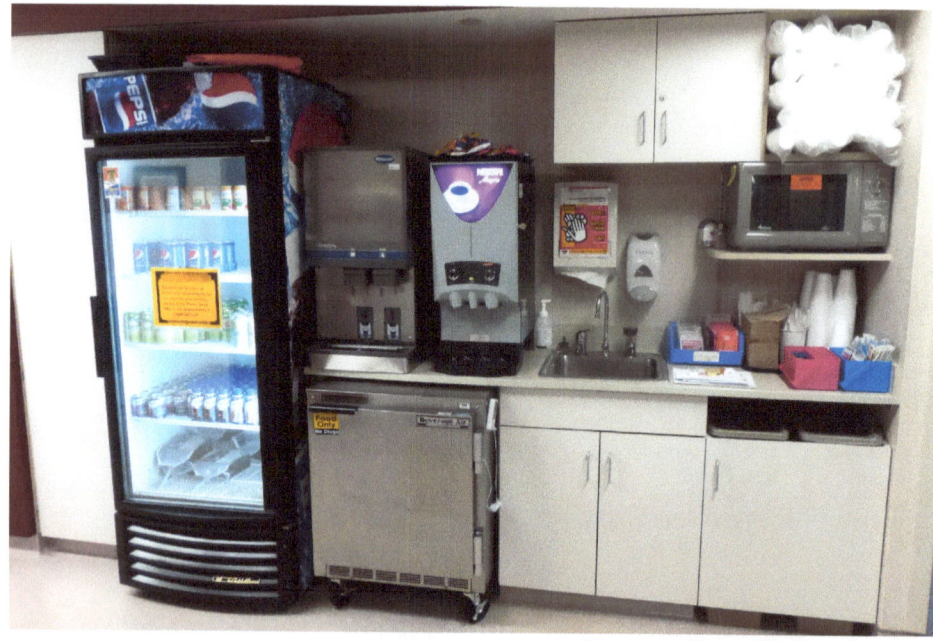

Chemotherapy = Systematic Runs throughout body

"Chemotherapy is a drug treatment that uses powerful chemicals to kill fast-growing cells in your body."

"Many different chemotherapy drugs are available. Chemotherapy drugs can be used alone or in combination to treat a wide variety of cancers."

"You'll meet with your cancer doctor (oncologist) regularly during chemotherapy treatment. Your oncologist will ask about any side effects you're experiencing, since many can be controlled."

"Depending on your situation, you may also undergo scans and other tests to monitor your cancer during chemotherapy treatment. These tests can give your doctor an idea of how your cancer is responding to treatment, and your treatment may be adjusted accordingly."

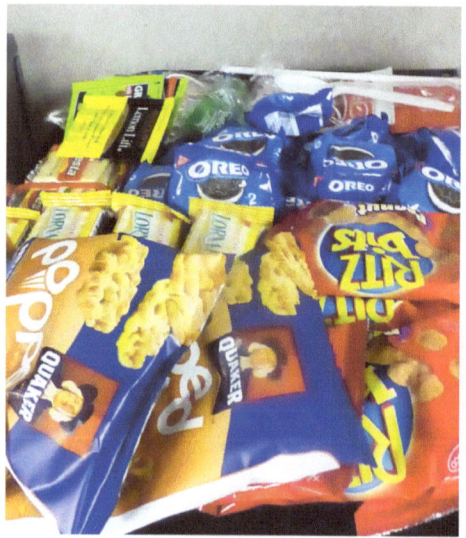
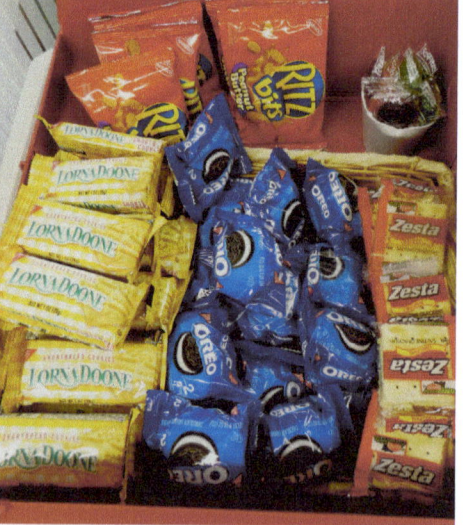

Chemotherapy Department Snacks
Gonda Building - 10 East

Radiation = Localized
Cleans up any cancerous "seeds" leftover from the chemo that may be too small to be detected.

"Radiation therapy is a type of cancer treatment that uses beams of intense energy to kill cancer cells. Radiation therapy most often gets its power from X-rays, but the power can also come from protons or other types of energy."

"The term "radiation therapy" most often refers to external beam radiation therapy. During this type of radiation, the high-energy beams come from a machine outside of your body that aims the beams at a precise point on your body. During a different type of radiation treatment called brachytherapy (brak-e-THER-uh-pee), radiation is placed inside your body."

"Radiation therapy damages cells by destroying the genetic material that controls how cells grow and divide. While both healthy and cancerous cells are damaged by radiation therapy, the goal of radiation therapy is to destroy as few normal, healthy cells as possible."

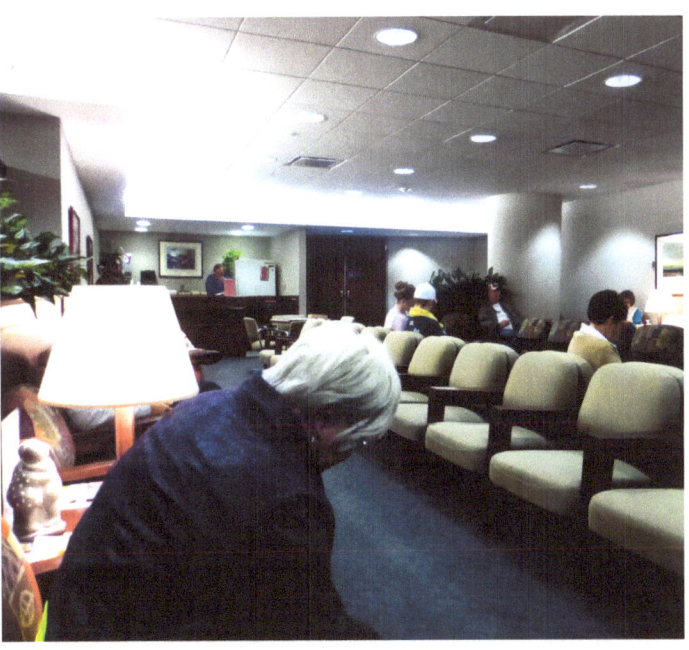

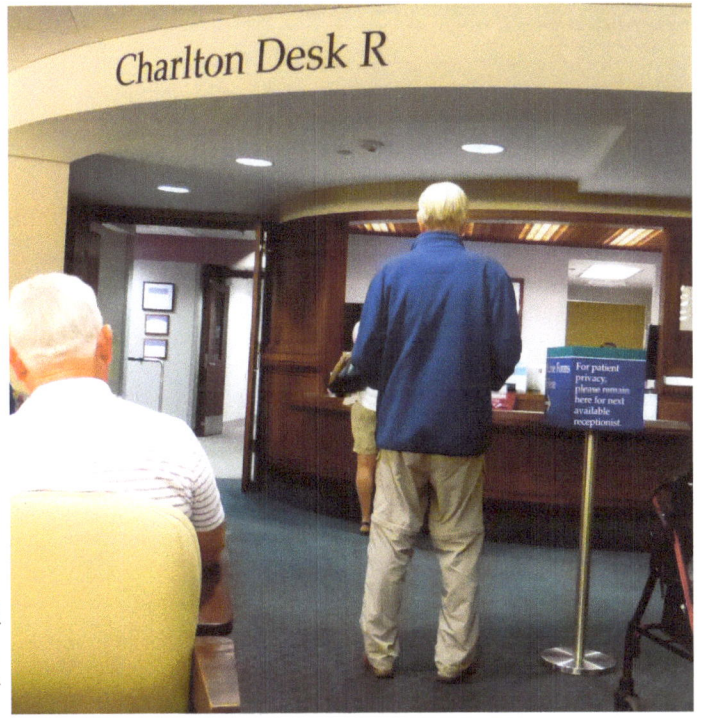

Radiation Waiting Room
Charlton Building - Desk R

Mayo Clinic Doctors & Appointments

12/30/2013 Medical Oncology Supervisory Ruddy, Kathryn Jean, MD

12/30/2013 Medical Oncology Consult Olson, Emily Anne, MSN, RN, CNP

01/07/2014 Radiation Oncology Supervisory Childs, Stephanie Krejcarek, MD

01/07/2014 Radiation Oncology Consult Rollmann, Denise Claire, RN, CNP

01/07/2014 General Surgery Consult Jakub, James W, MD

01/10/2014 Medical Oncology Subsequent Visit Olson, Emily Anne, MSN, RN, CNP

01/10/2014 Diagnostic Radiology Assessment Maurer, Mindy Rene, RN

01/20/2014 Cardiovascular Consult Rodeheffer, Richard J, MD

01/29/2014 Medical Oncology Test Only Miscellaneous Olson, Emily Anne, MSN, RN, CNP

02/10/2014 Medical Oncology Subsequent Visit Olson, Emily Anne, MSN, RN, CNP

02/10/2014 Diagnostic Radiology Assessment Steele, Amanda Jo

02/10/2014 Direct Hospital Admit Referral Misc Jahns, Nicole Marie, RN

02/10/2014 Hospital Admission Note Sharain, Korosh, MD

02/10/2014 Hospital Admission Note Larsen, Jeremy Todd, MD

02/11/2014 Discharge Planning Kyllo, Dawn Marie, MS, RN

02/11/2014 Hospital Admission Note Costello, Brian A, MD

02/11/2014 Respiratory Therapy Bogenrief, Angela Mary, RRT

02/12/2014 Hospital Summary Costello, Brian A, MD

02/14/2014 Medical Oncology Miscellaneous Olson, Emily Anne, MSN, RN, CNP

02/24/2014 Medical Oncology Subsequent Visit Olson, Emily Anne, MSN, RN, CNP

03/03/2014 Thrombophilia Consult Ransone, Teresa R, PA-C

03/24/2014 Medical Oncology Subsequent Visit Ruddy, Kathryn Jean, MD

03/31/2014 Thrombophilia Subsequent Visit Ransone, Teresa R, PA-C

04/14/2014 Oncology Therapy Maschka, Jennifer Lynn, RN

04/14/2014 Womens Heart Consult Mulvagh, Sharon Lee, MD

04/21/2014 Medical Oncology Subsequent Visit Ruddy, Kathryn Jean, MD

05/05/2014 Medical Oncology Subsequent Visit Ruddy, Kathryn Jean, MD

05/19/2014 Medical Oncology Subsequent Visit Chintakuntlawar, Ashish Vitthalrao, MBBS, PhD

05/20/2014 Physical Medicine & Rehabilitation Con Hanson, Toni J, MD

06/02/2014 Medical Oncology Subsequent Visit Chintakuntlawar, Ashish Vitthalrao, MBBS, PhD

06/03/2014 Oncology Therapy Spohn, Jeraldine Kay Lee, RN

06/09/2014 Radiation Oncology Supervisory Childs, Stephanie Krejcarek, MD

06/09/2014 Radiation Oncology Subsequent Visit Rollmann, Denise Claire, RN, CNP

06/10/2014 Radiation Oncology Miscellaneous Childs, Stephanie Krejcarek, MD

06/24/2014 Radiation Oncology Therapy Schultz, Carolyn J, RN

06/25/2014 Radiation Oncology Therapy Rollmann, Denise Claire, RN, CNP

07/02/2014 Radiation Oncology Therapy Childs, Stephanie Krejcarek, MD

07/02/2014 Radiation Oncology Therapy Hardie, John G, MD, PhD

07/08/2014 Radiation Oncology Therapy Hardie, John G, MD, PhD

07/10/2014 Radiation Oncology Therapy Schultz, Carolyn J, RN

07/15/2014 Radiation Oncology Therapy Hardie, John G, MD, PhD

07/17/2014 Radiation Oncology Therapy Schultz, Carolyn J, RN

07/22/2014 Radiation Oncology Therapy Hardie, John G, MD, PhD

07/24/2014 Radiation Oncology Therapy Schultz, Carolyn J, RN

07/29/2014 Radiation Oncology Therapy Hardie, John G, MD, PhD

07/30/2014 Radiation Oncology Therapy Schultz, Carolyn J, RN

07/30/2014 Thrombophilia Consult Jennings, Lea B, RN, CNP

08/04/2014 Radiation Oncology Therapy Schultz, Carolyn J, RN

Timeline

July 22, 2013
Had Mammogram.

August 20, 2013
Received news that the lump was malignant, Stage 3 Aggressive Breast Cancer.

August 21, 2013
First surgery (out-patient) to remove five-centimeter lump in Fosston, Minnesota.
Tumor was the size of a golf ball or larger.
Dr. Robert Wrobleuski was the surgeon for all three procedures in Fosston.

September 18, 2013
Second surgery to take a biopsy of the right breast in Fosston.
Sentinel Lymph Node was removed and tested.
Spent the night at the hospital.

November 13, 2013
Third surgery (out-patient) in Fosston to clean-up margins around where cancerous tumors had been present.

January 13, 2014 - June 2, 2014
Sixteen weekly chemotherapy treatments.
Twelve Taxol Chemotherapy & Four E.C. Chemotherapy treatments.

February 10, 2014 - February 12, 2014
Hospitalized with Pulmonary Embolism Blood Clots at Mayo Clinic Methodist Hospital.

June 9 , 2014
Ultrasound of breast.
Good news: "No cancer in lymph nodes."

June 23, 2014 - August 4, 2014
Six weeks of thirty radiation treatments.

All Walks of Life in Rochester

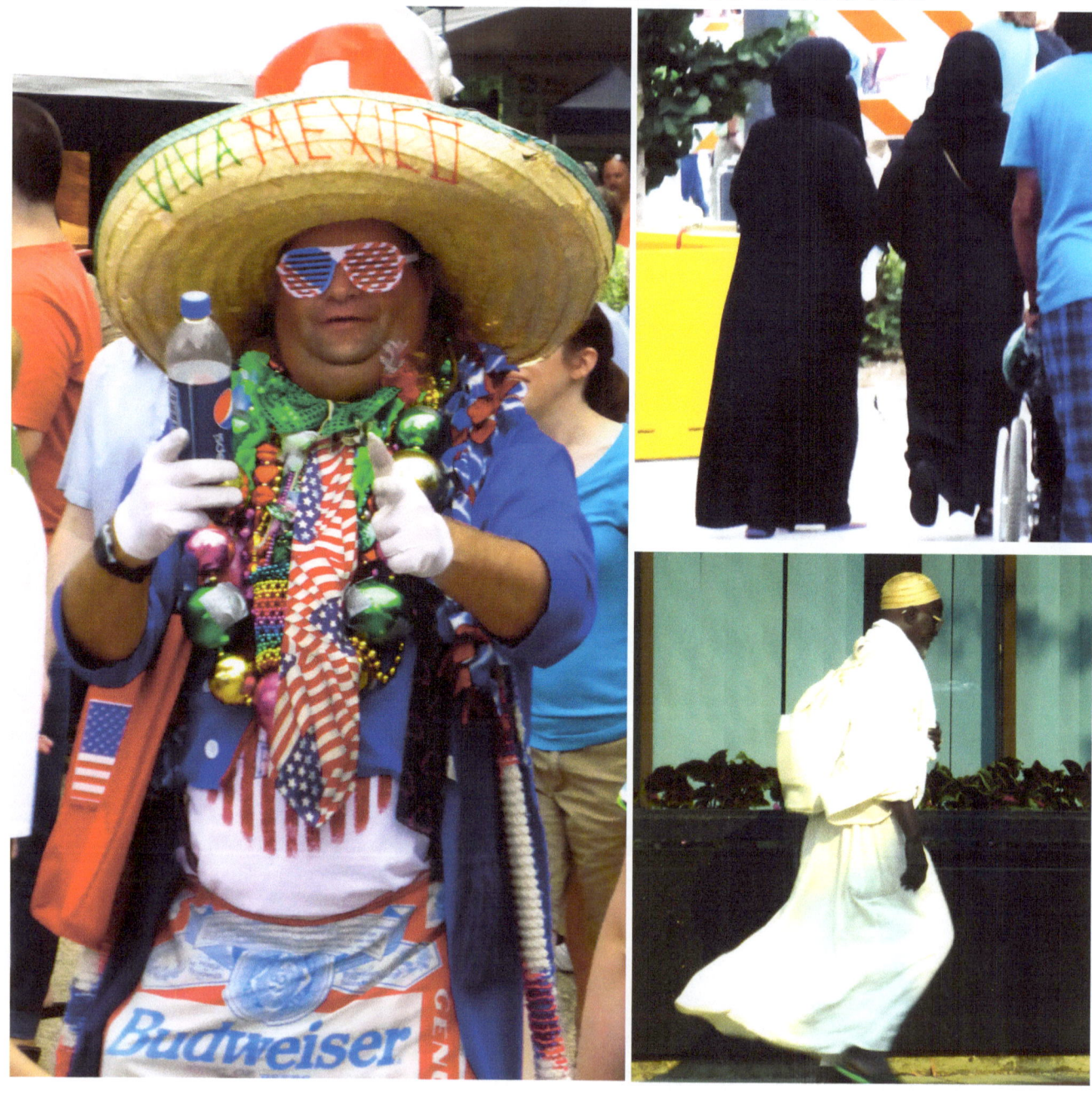

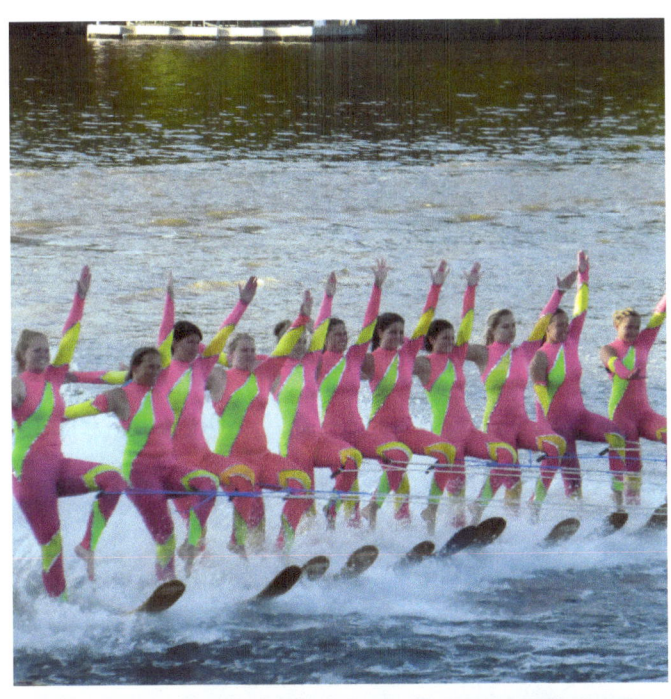

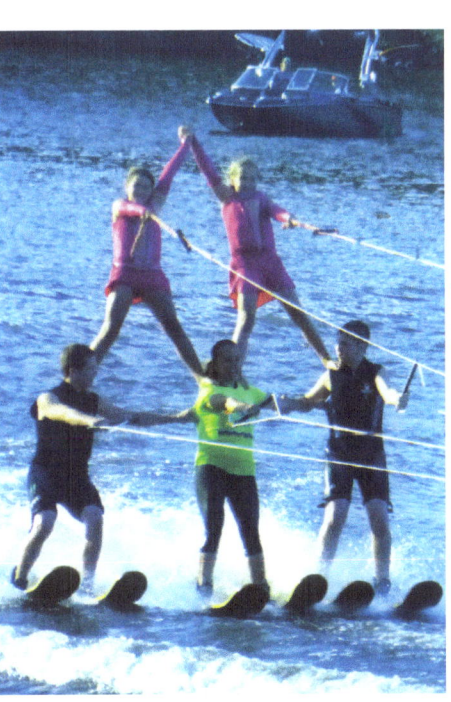

SkiDox
Water
Ski
Show

Lake
Zumbro

Oronco,
Minnesota

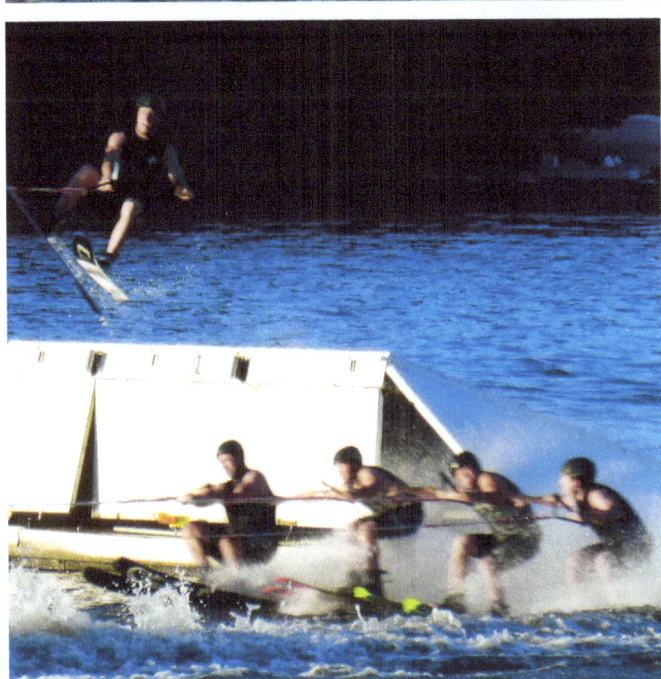

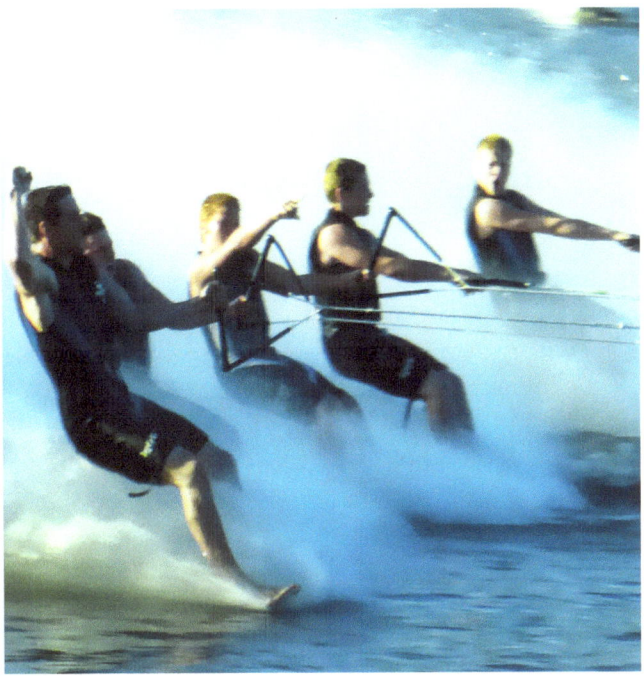

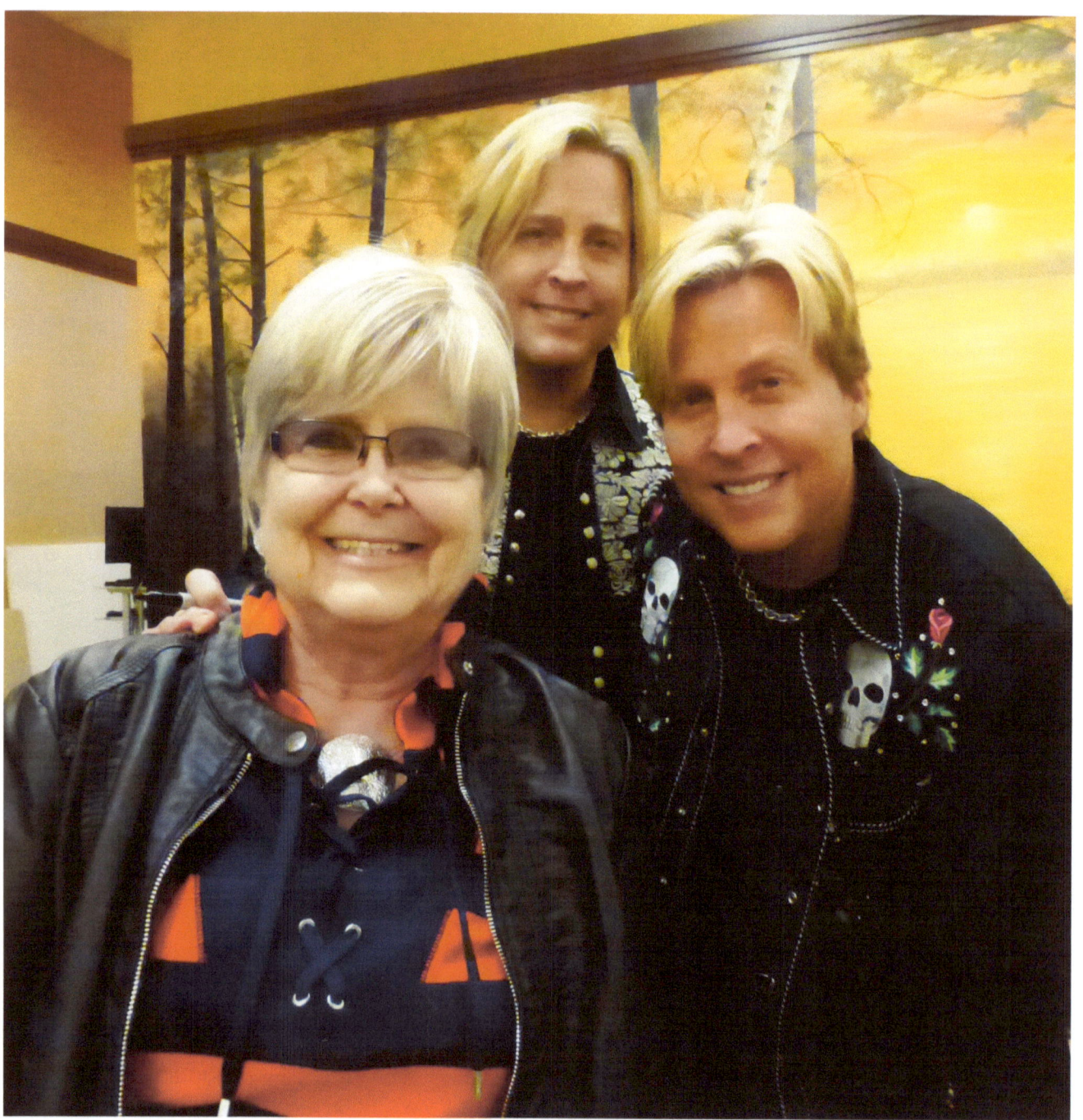

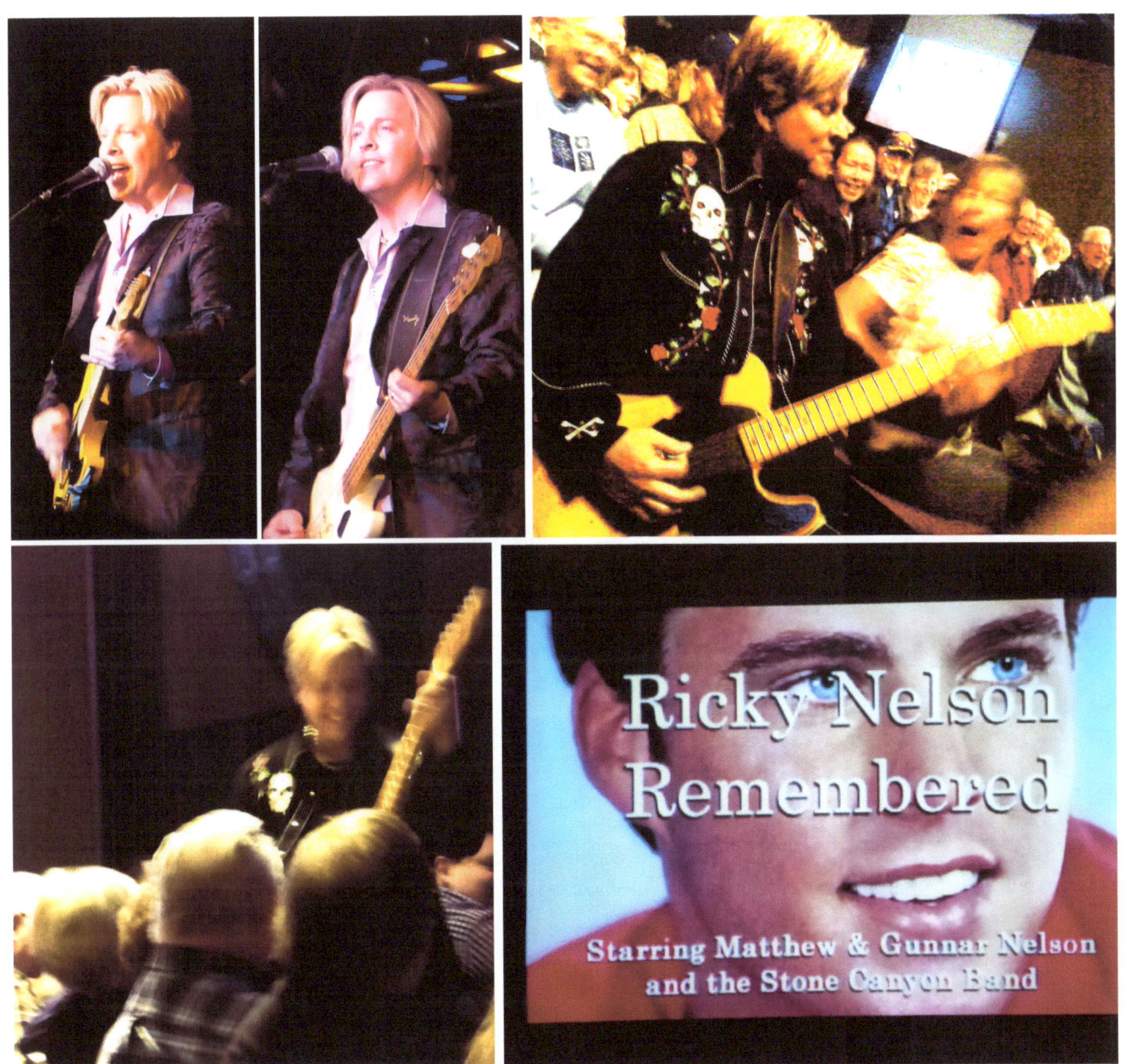

Ricky Nelson
Remembered

Starring Matthew & Gunnar Nelson
and the Stone Canyon Band

Ricky Nelson Tribute Concert in Walker
Matthew & Gunnar Nelson

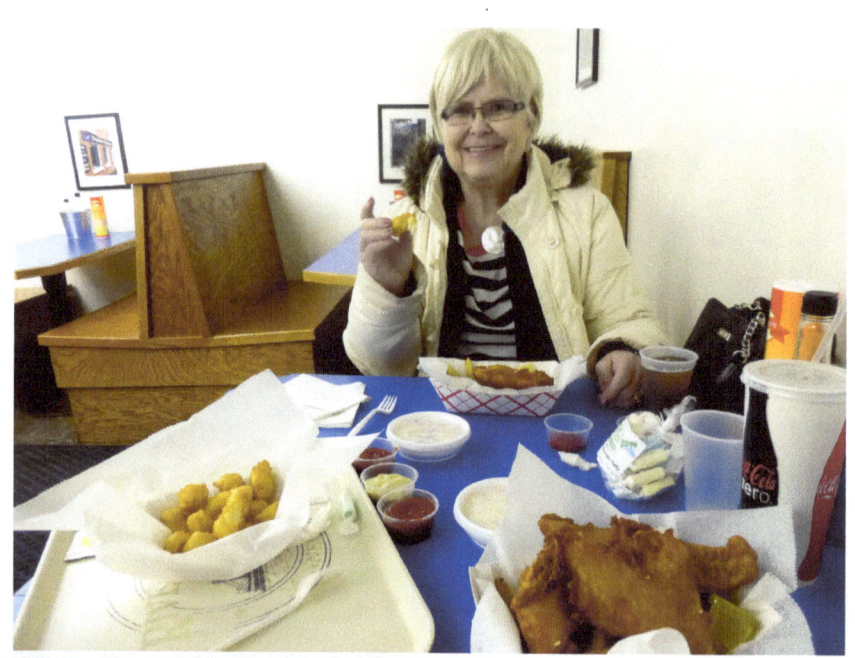

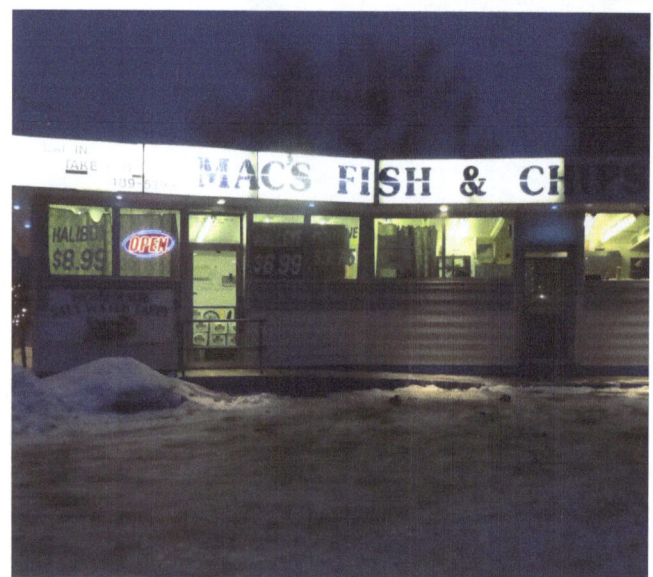

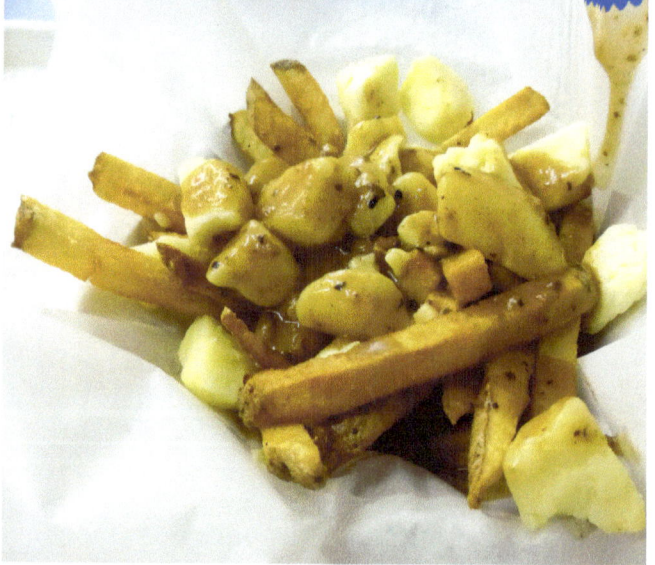

Mac's Fish & Chips
St. Paul, Minnesota
Poutine (bottom-right): French Fries, Brown Gravy, & Cheese Curds.

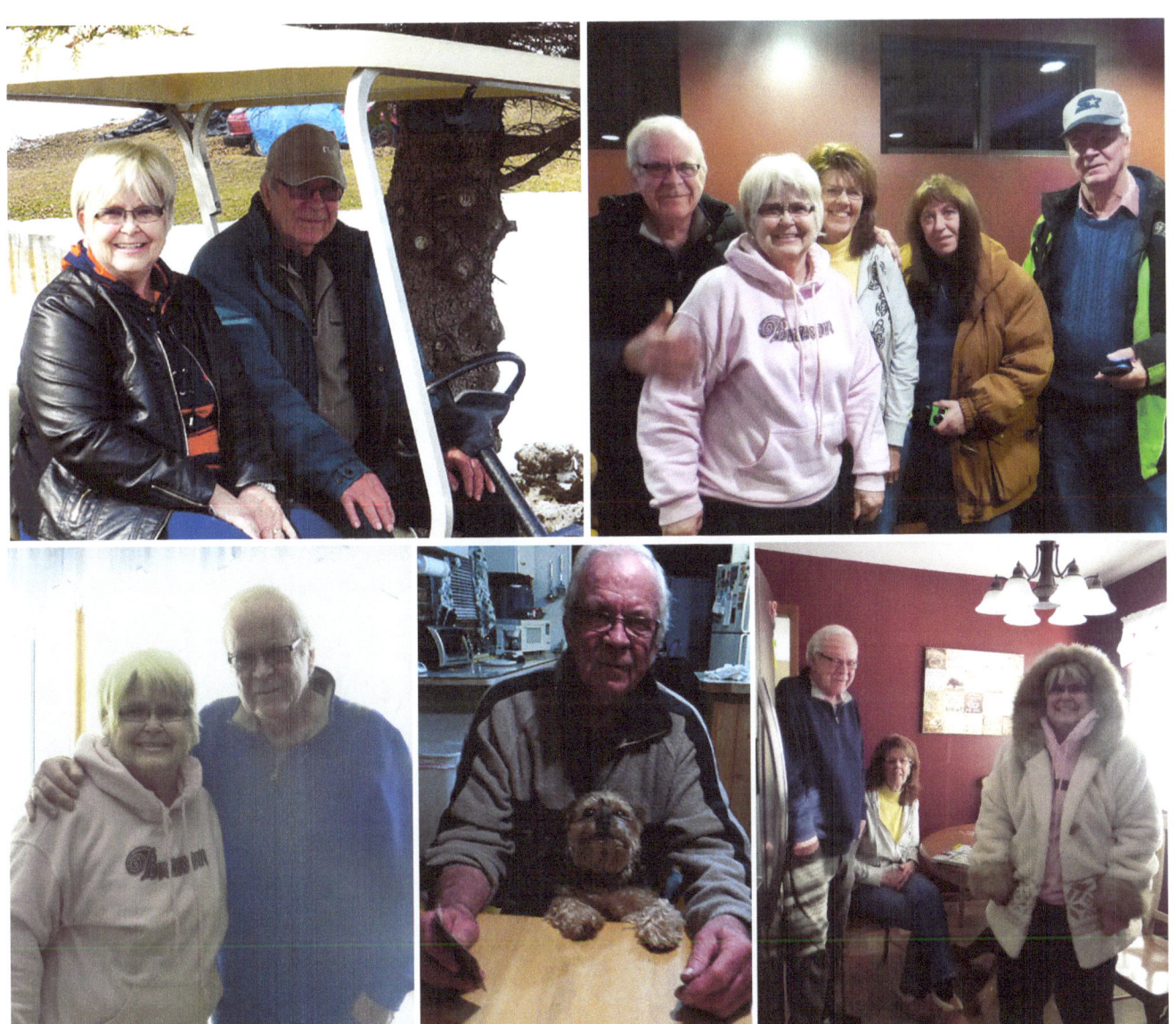

Staying With Larry

My brother Larry opened up his home to us, breaking our seven-hour drive to the Mayo nearly in half. What a good chance to also get to see and visit with my brother Lyle and his friend Charlotte. Larry would get up in the middle-of-the-night to make us breakfast and see us off. Visiting with Larry and Margaret may involve everything from catching-up with each other to puzzles to playing card games.

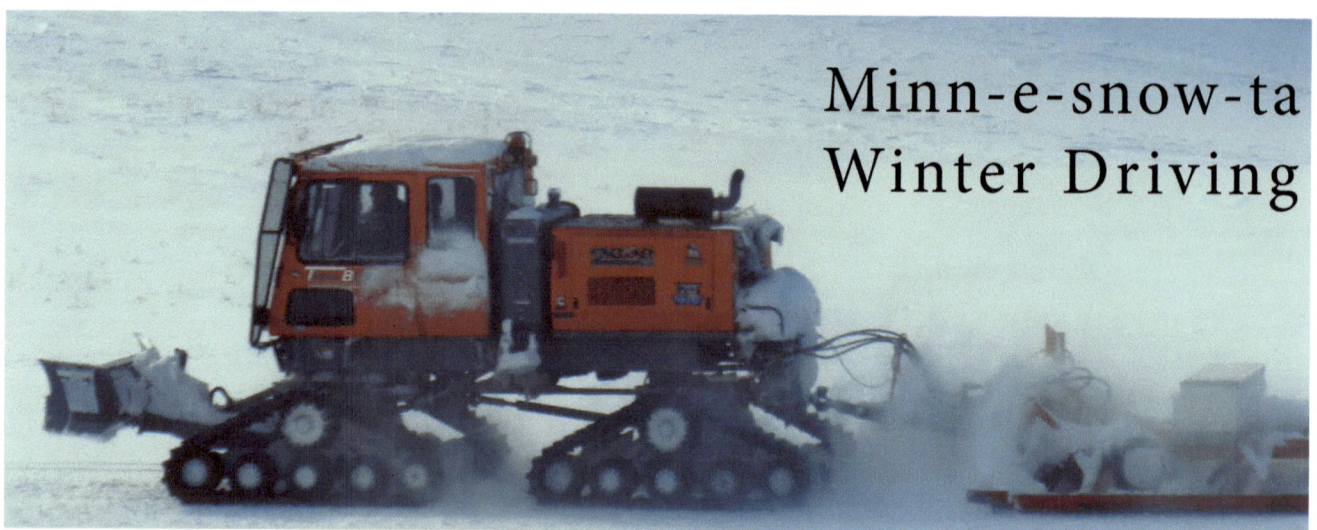

Minn-e-snow-ta Winter Driving

We were in all kinds of extreme weather. It was a tough, cold winter with lots of snow. One night it was -43 degrees F below when we left home, without counting the wind-chill. My water bottle froze in the car. It was common to have "No Travel Advisories" when the air temperature was -50 degrees F to -60 degrees F with the wind-chill. The outside temperature changed 69 degrees in exactly one week, from -28 degrees F one Sunday to 41 degrees F the next Sunday.

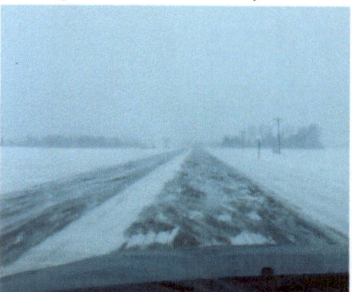
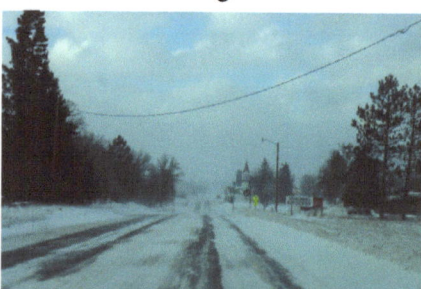
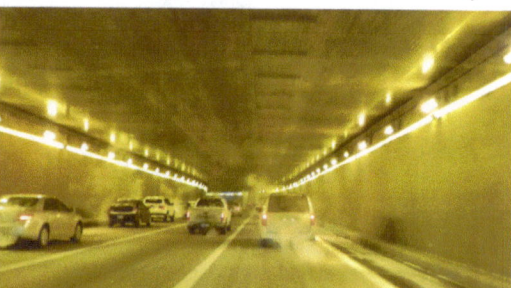

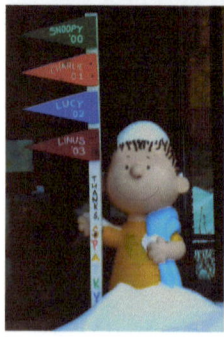
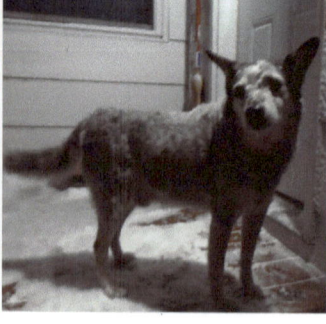
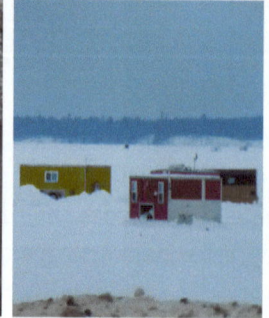
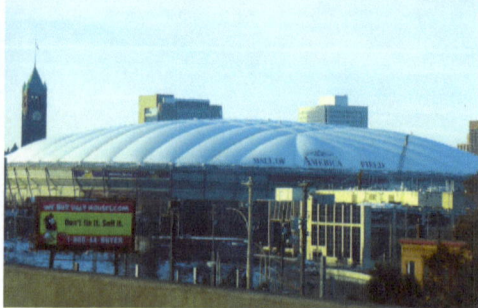

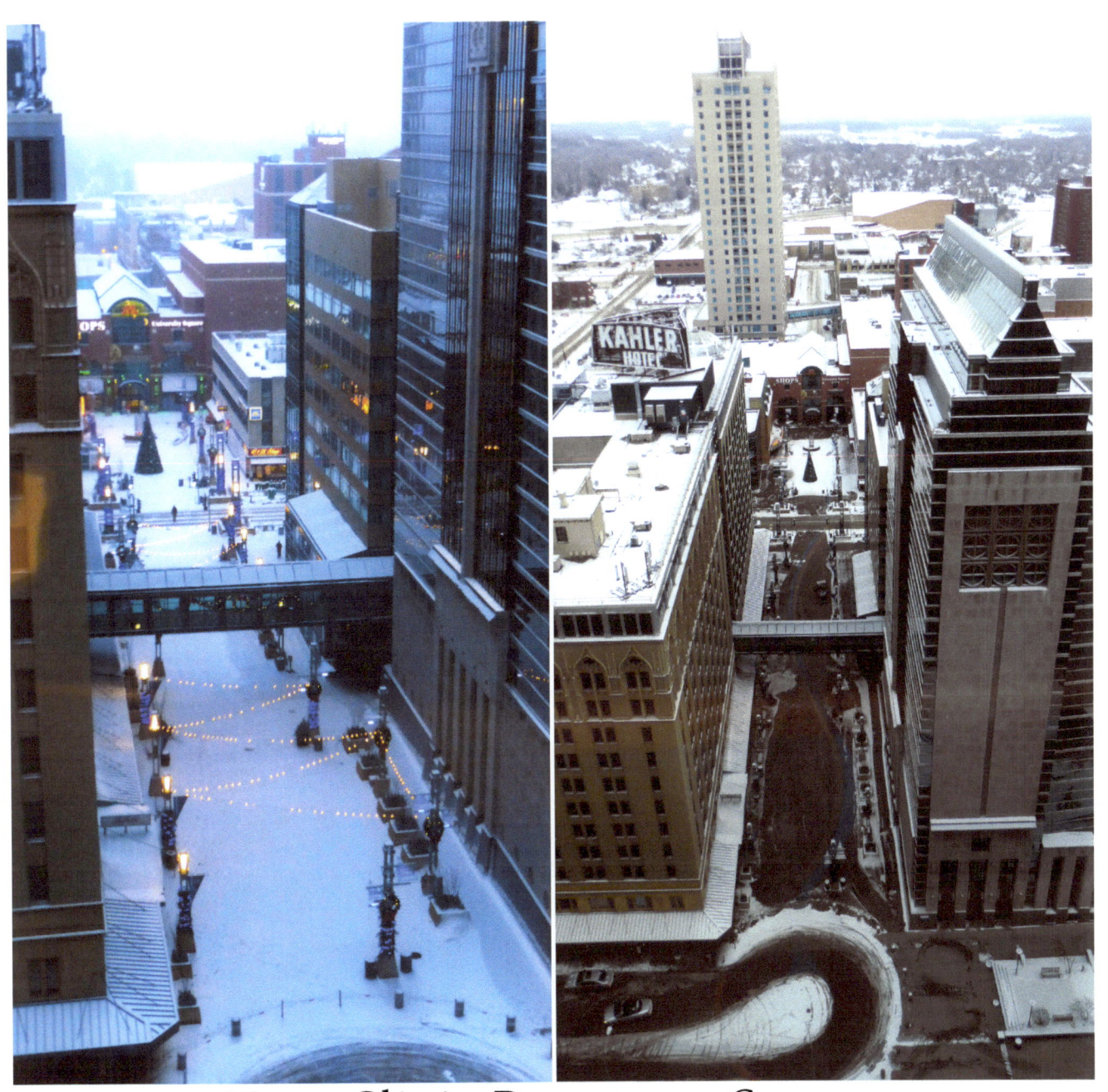

Mayo Clinic Downtown Campus

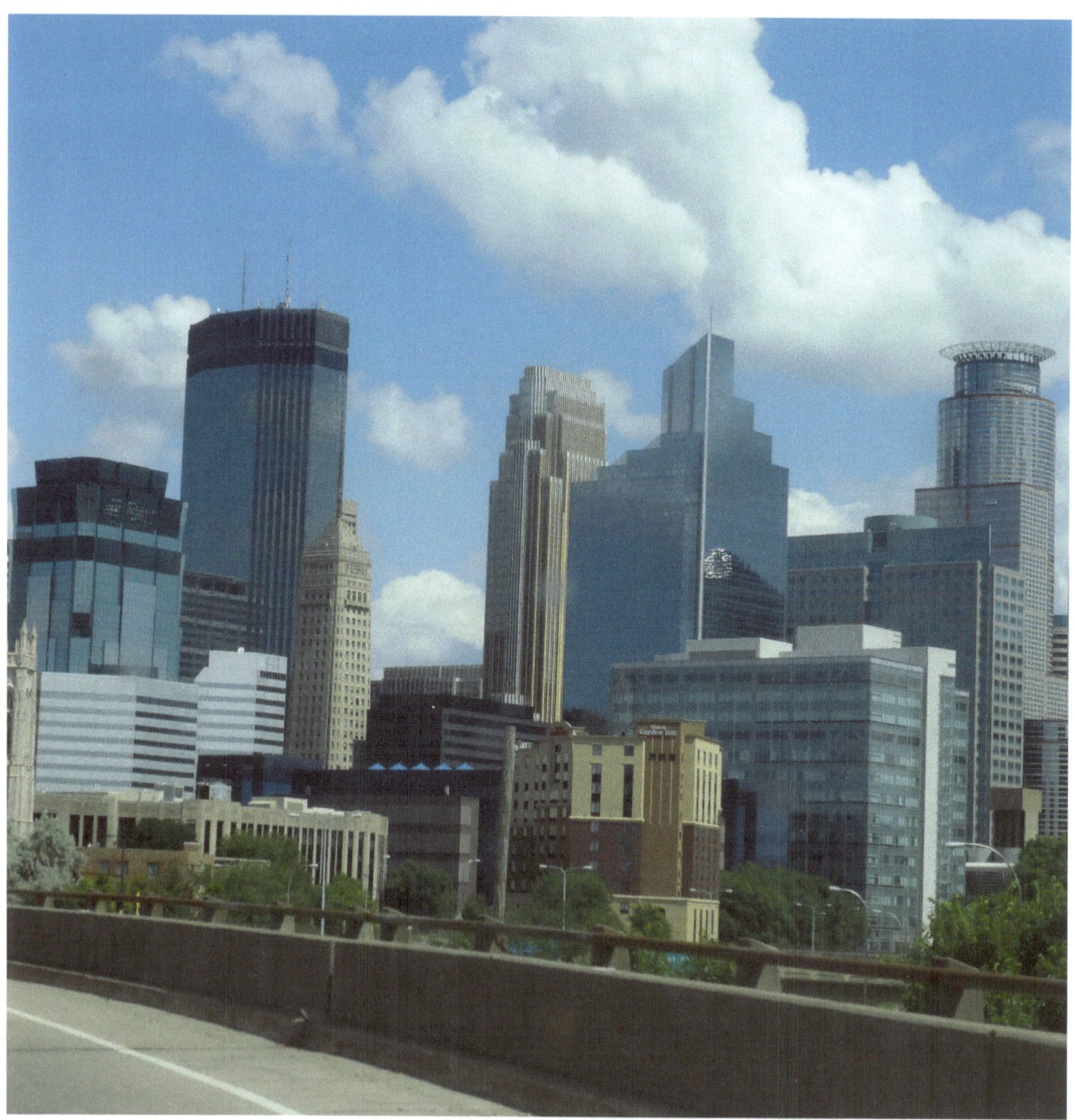

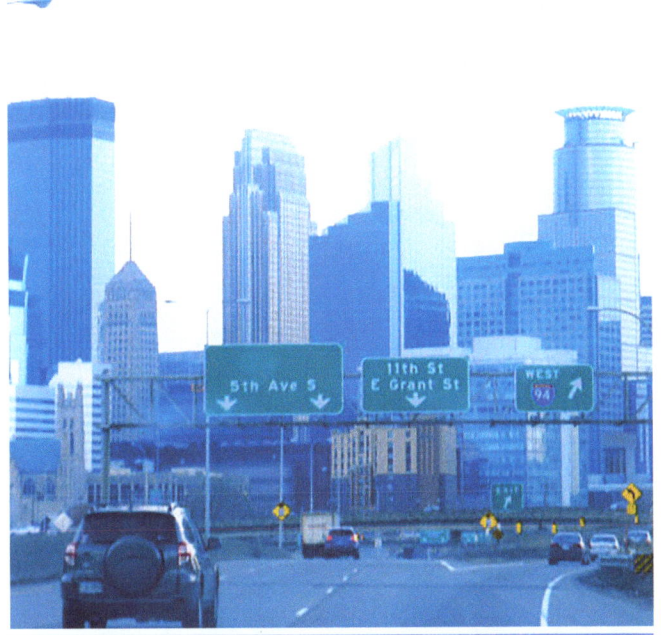

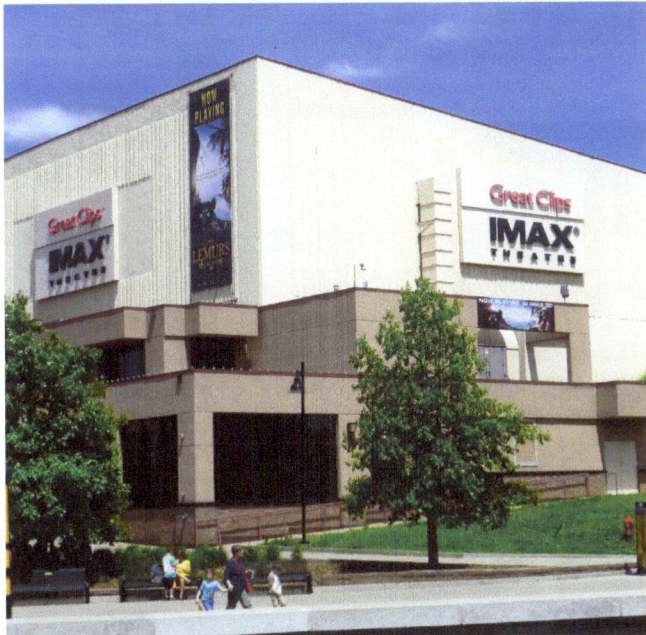

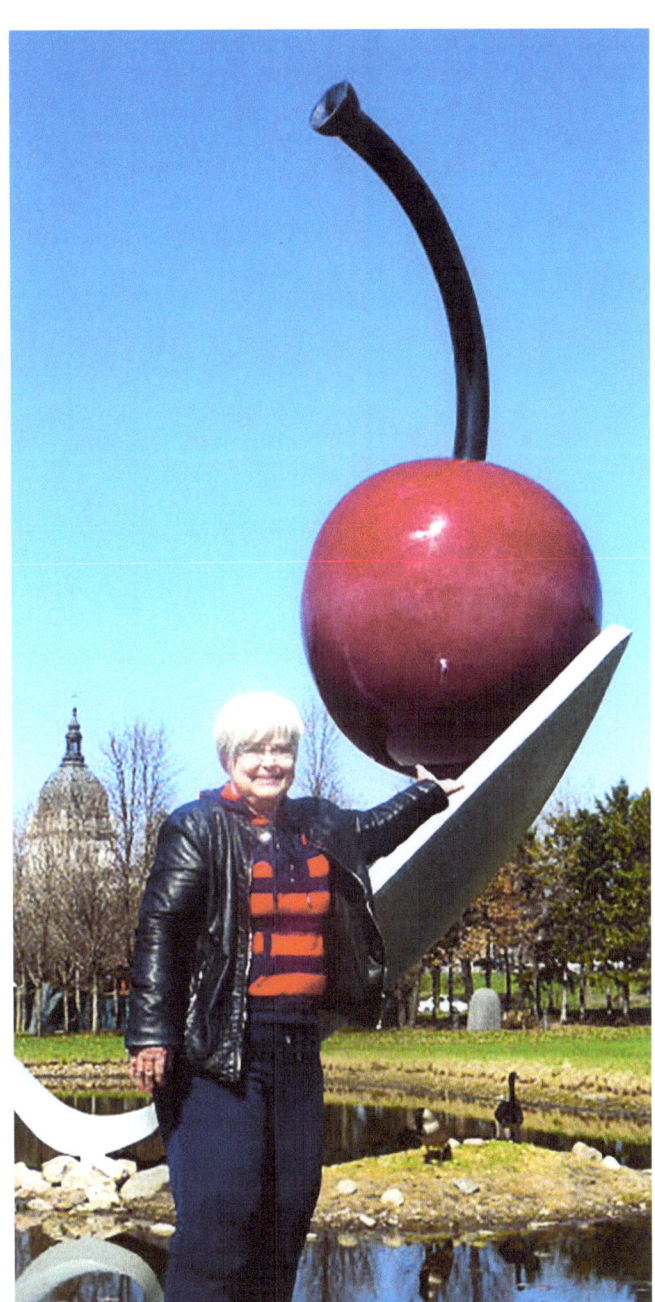

Minneapolis/St. Paul

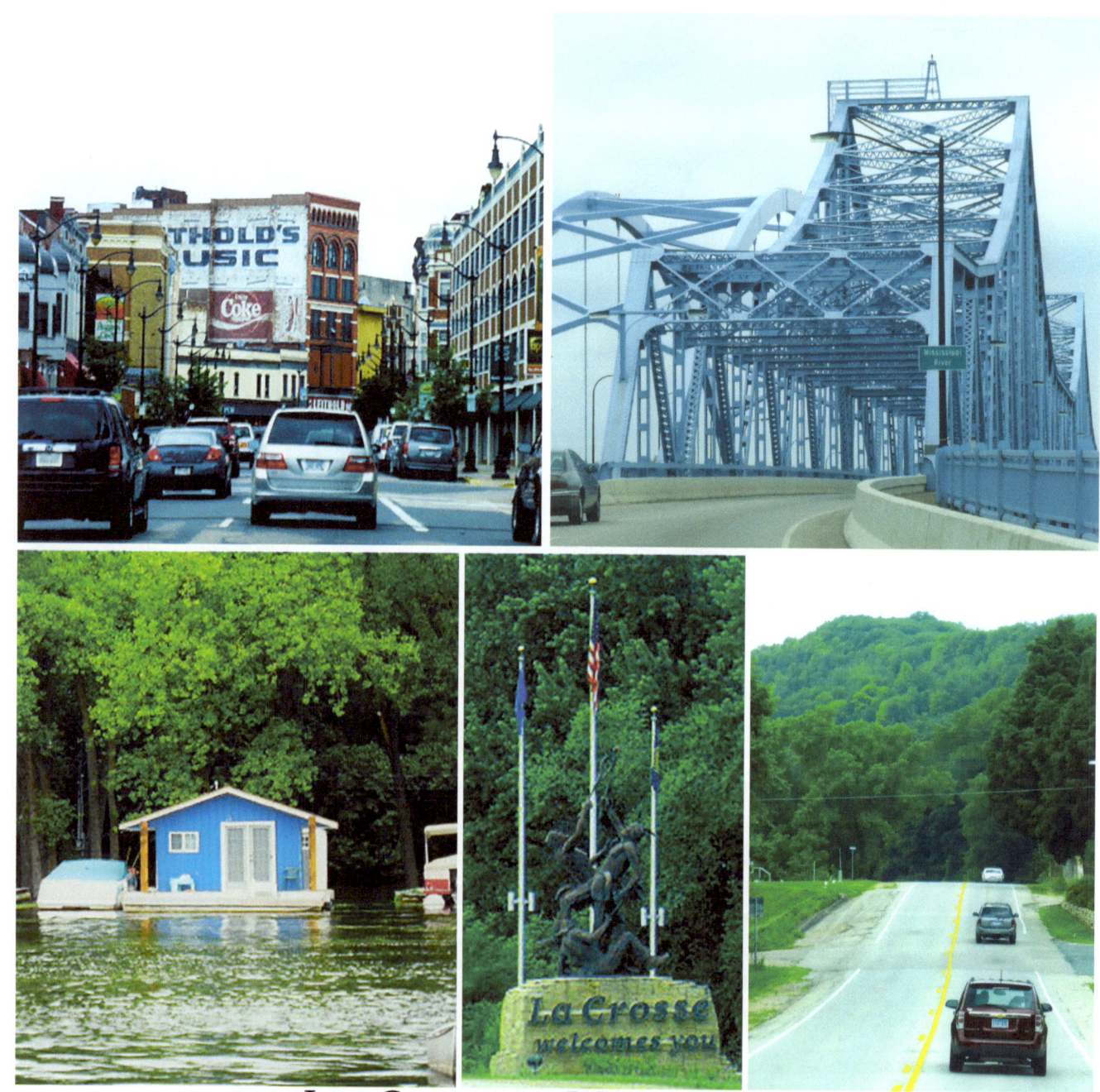

La Crosse, Wisconsin

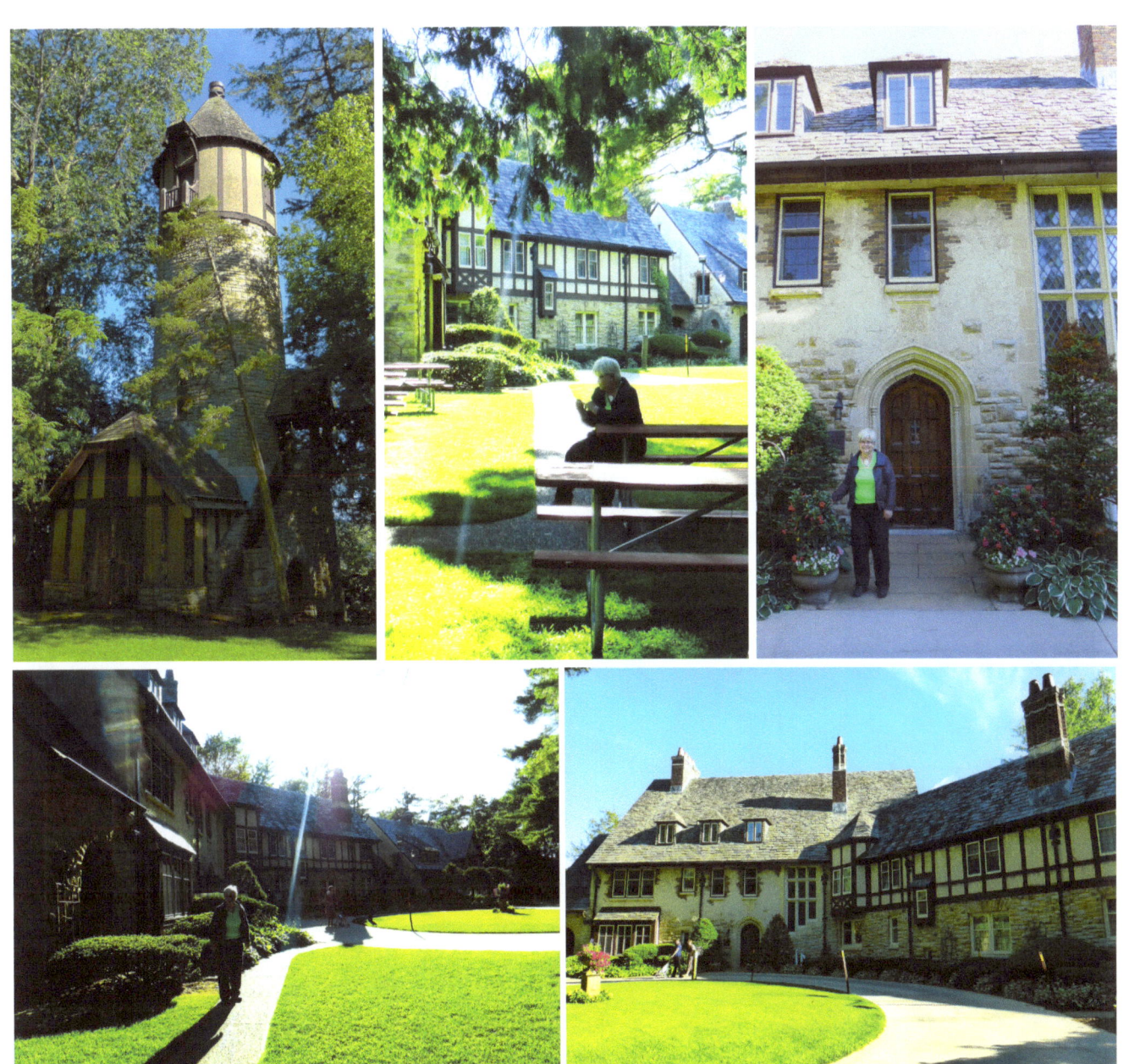

Plummer House
Rochester, Minnesota

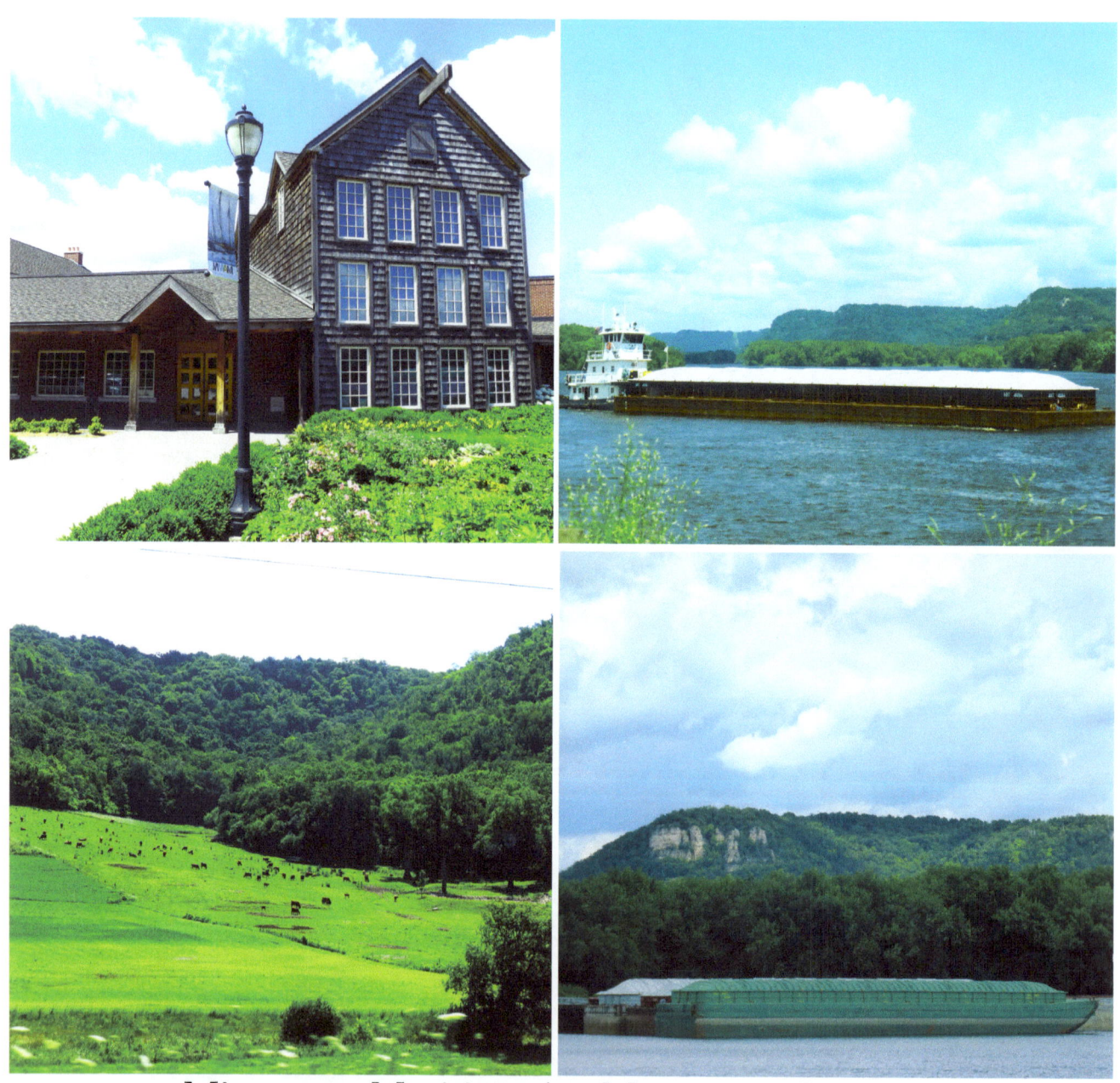

Minnesota Maritime Art Museum in Winona
Mississippi River Barges | Cattle Grazing in Caledonia, Minnesota

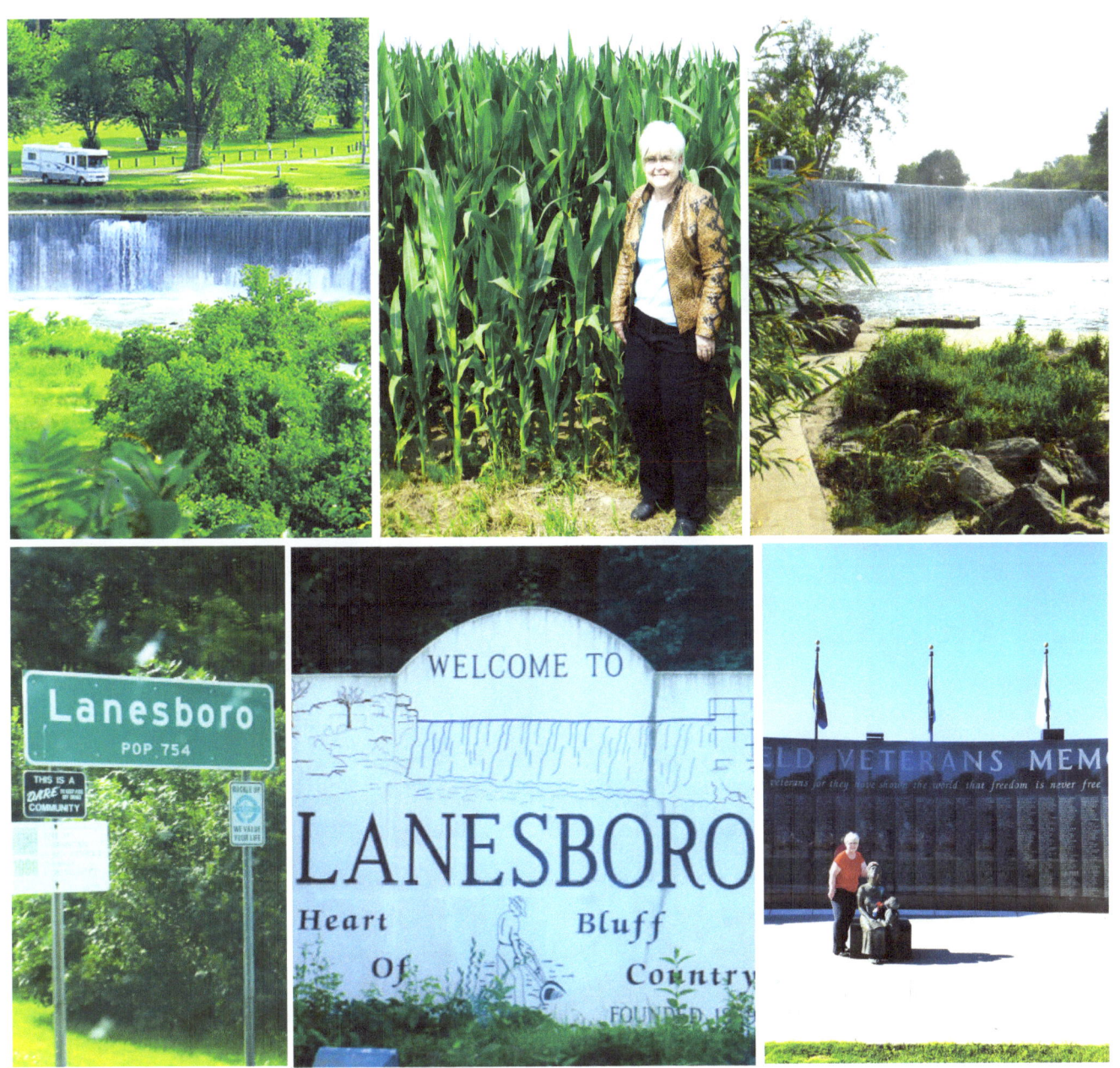

Lanesboro, Minnesota &
Veteran's Memorial in Rochester, Minnesota

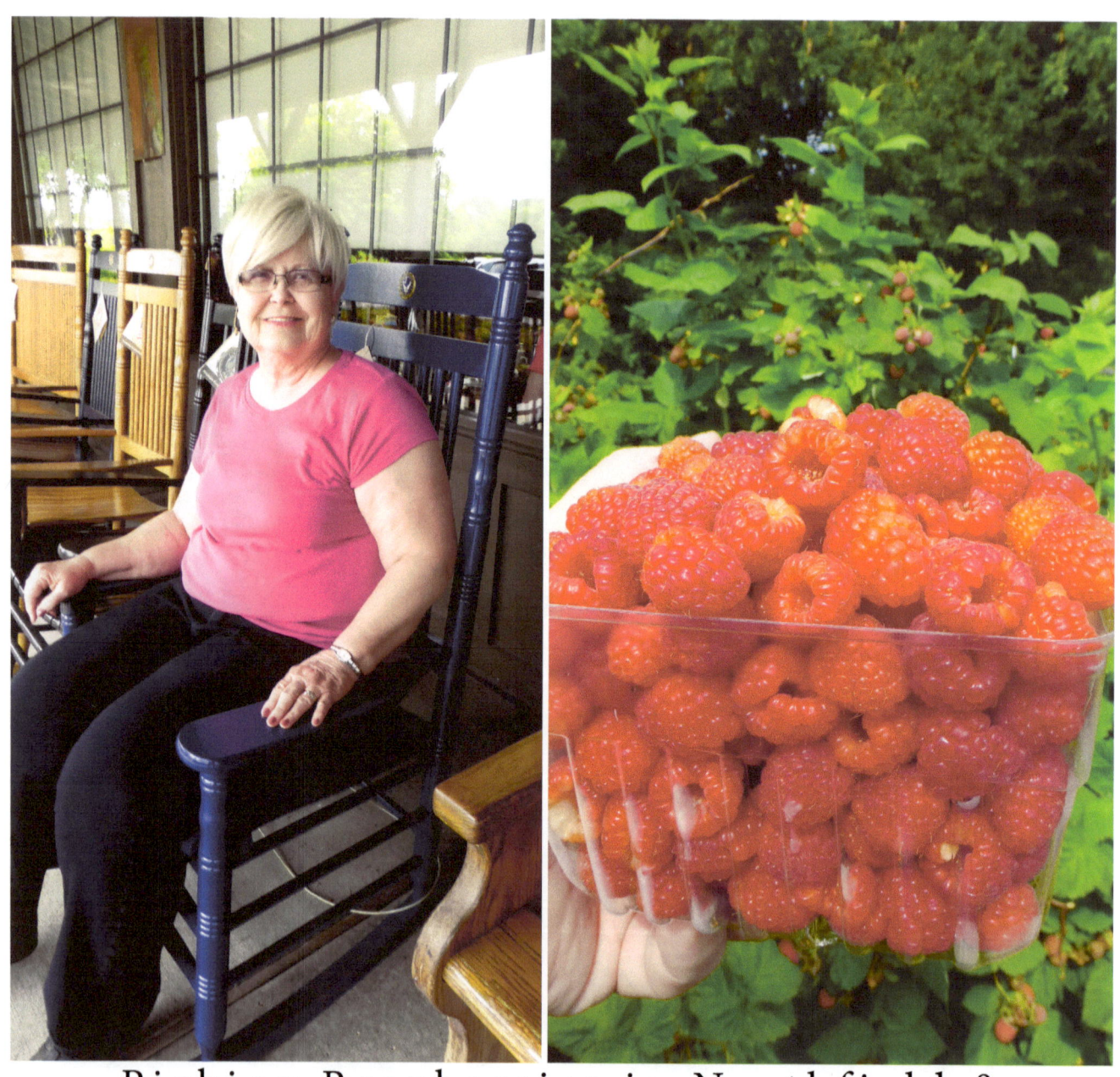

Picking Raspberries in Northfield &
Lunch at Cracker Barrel in Lakeville

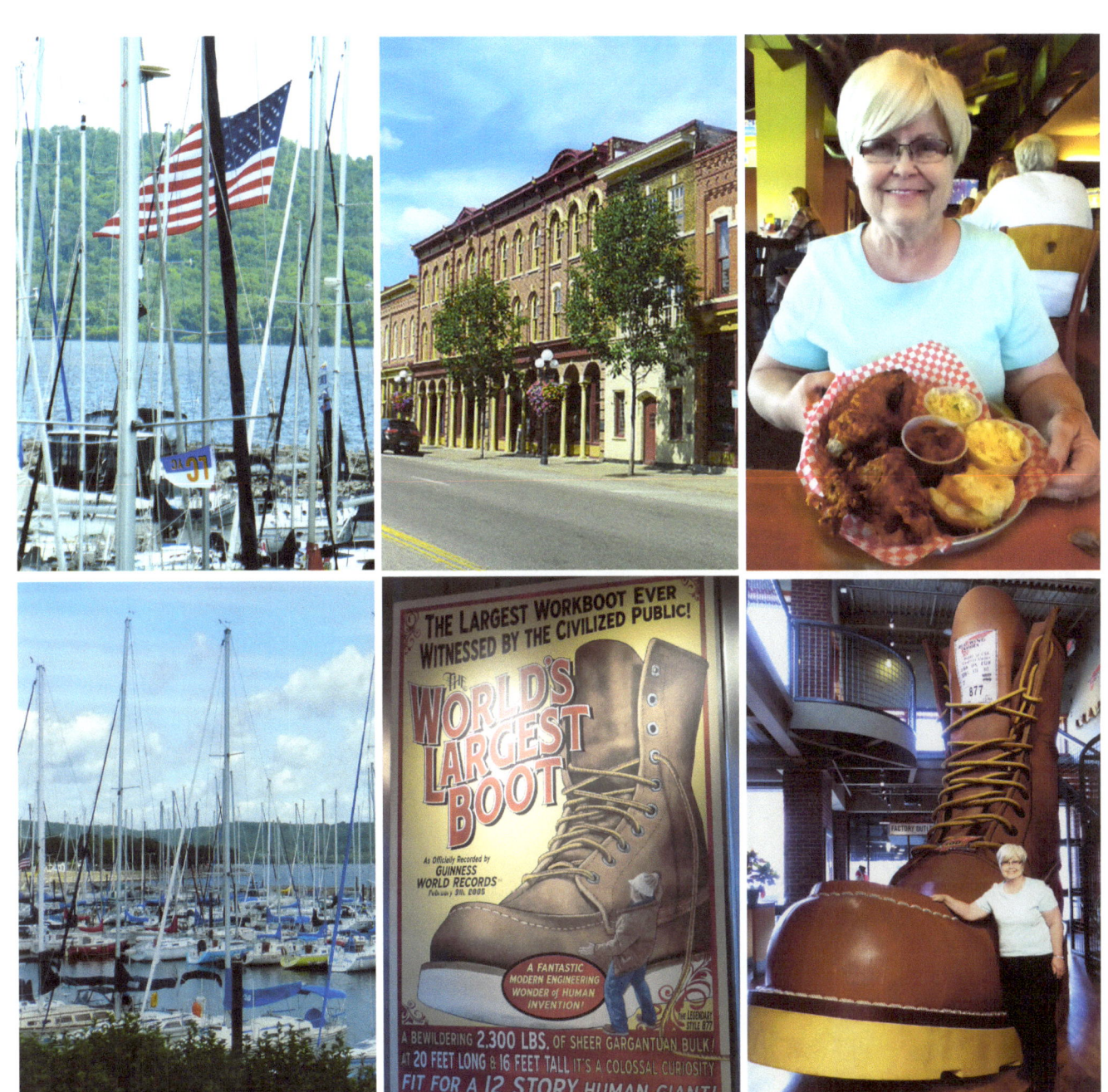

Red Wing & Lake City

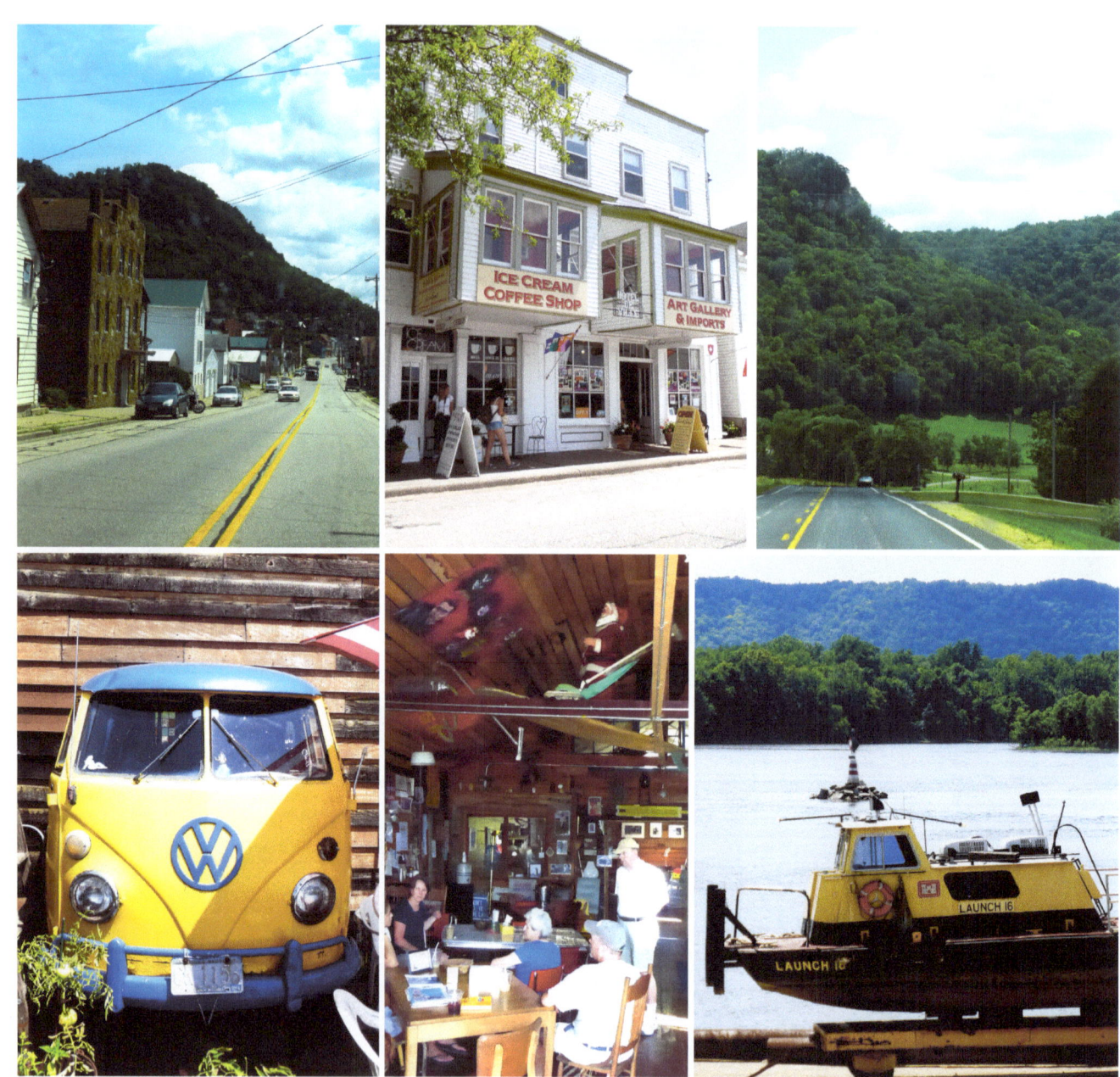

Bluff Country
Fountain City, Wisconsin

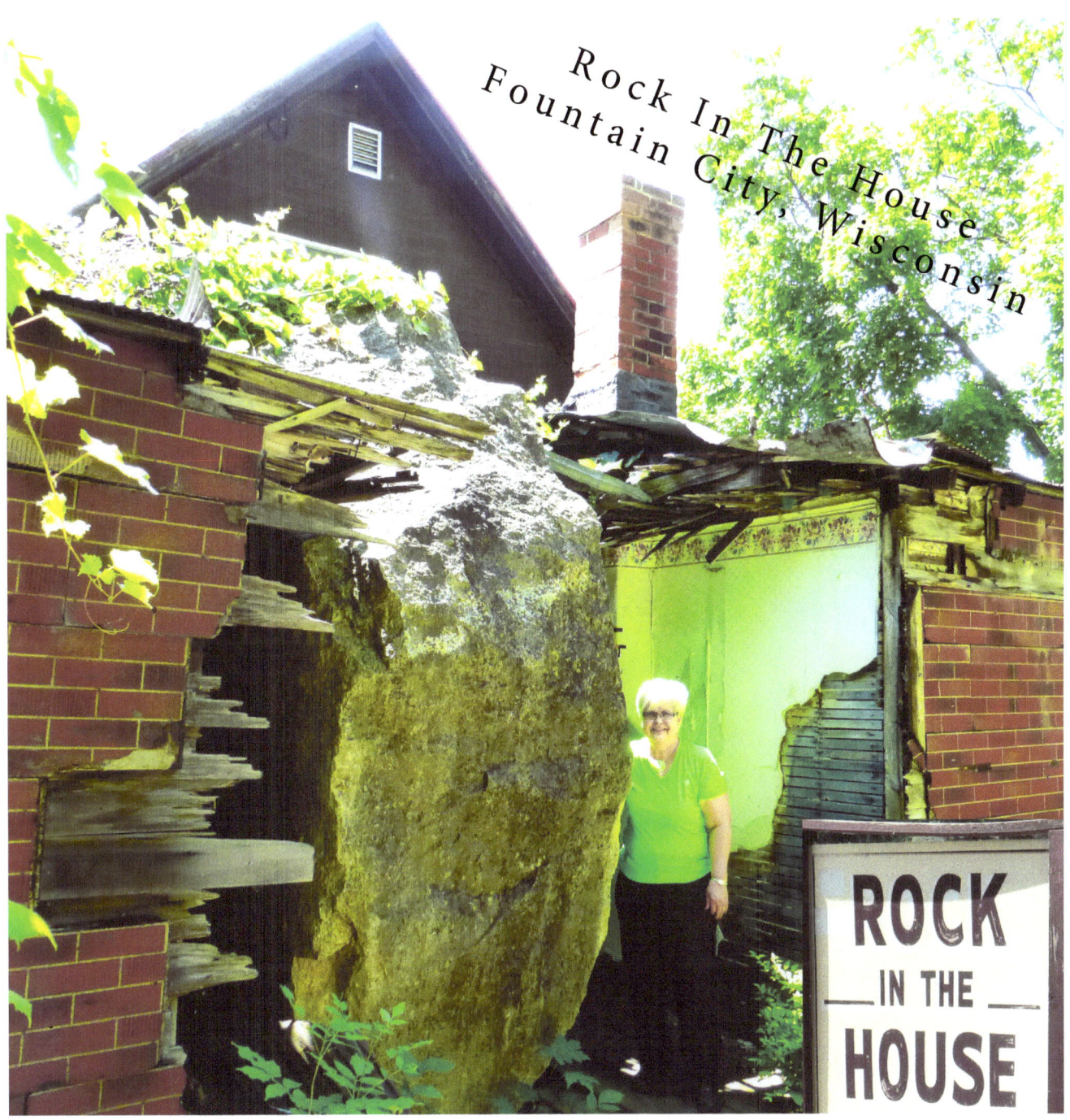

Rock In The House
Fountain City, Wisconsin

ROCK
IN THE
HOUSE

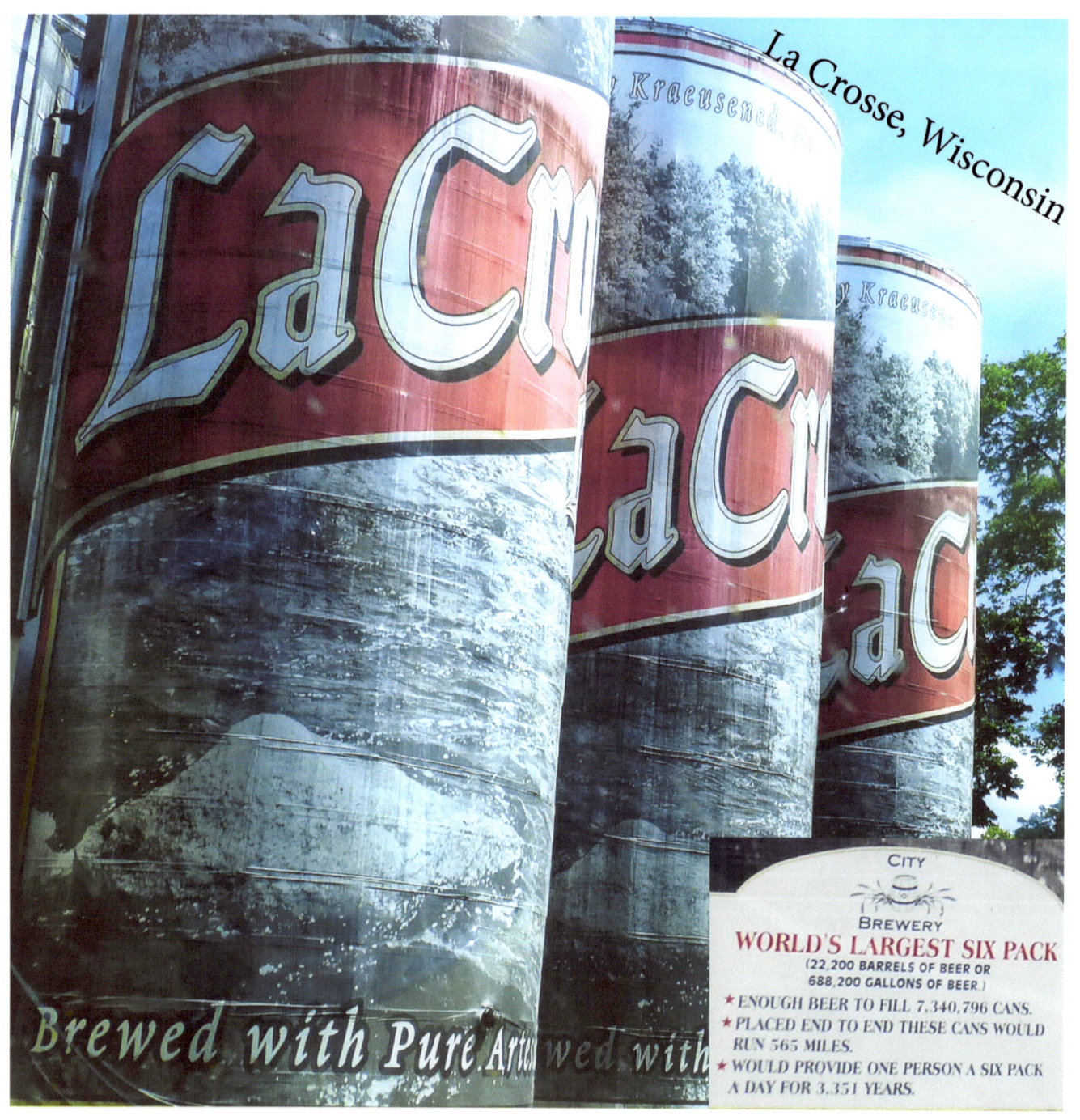

La Crosse, Wisconsin

CITY
BREWERY
WORLD'S LARGEST SIX PACK
(22,200 BARRELS OF BEER OR
688,200 GALLONS OF BEER.)

★ ENOUGH BEER TO FILL 7,340,796 CANS.
★ PLACED END TO END THESE CANS WOULD
RUN 565 MILES.
★ WOULD PROVIDE ONE PERSON A SIX PACK
A DAY FOR 3,351 YEARS.

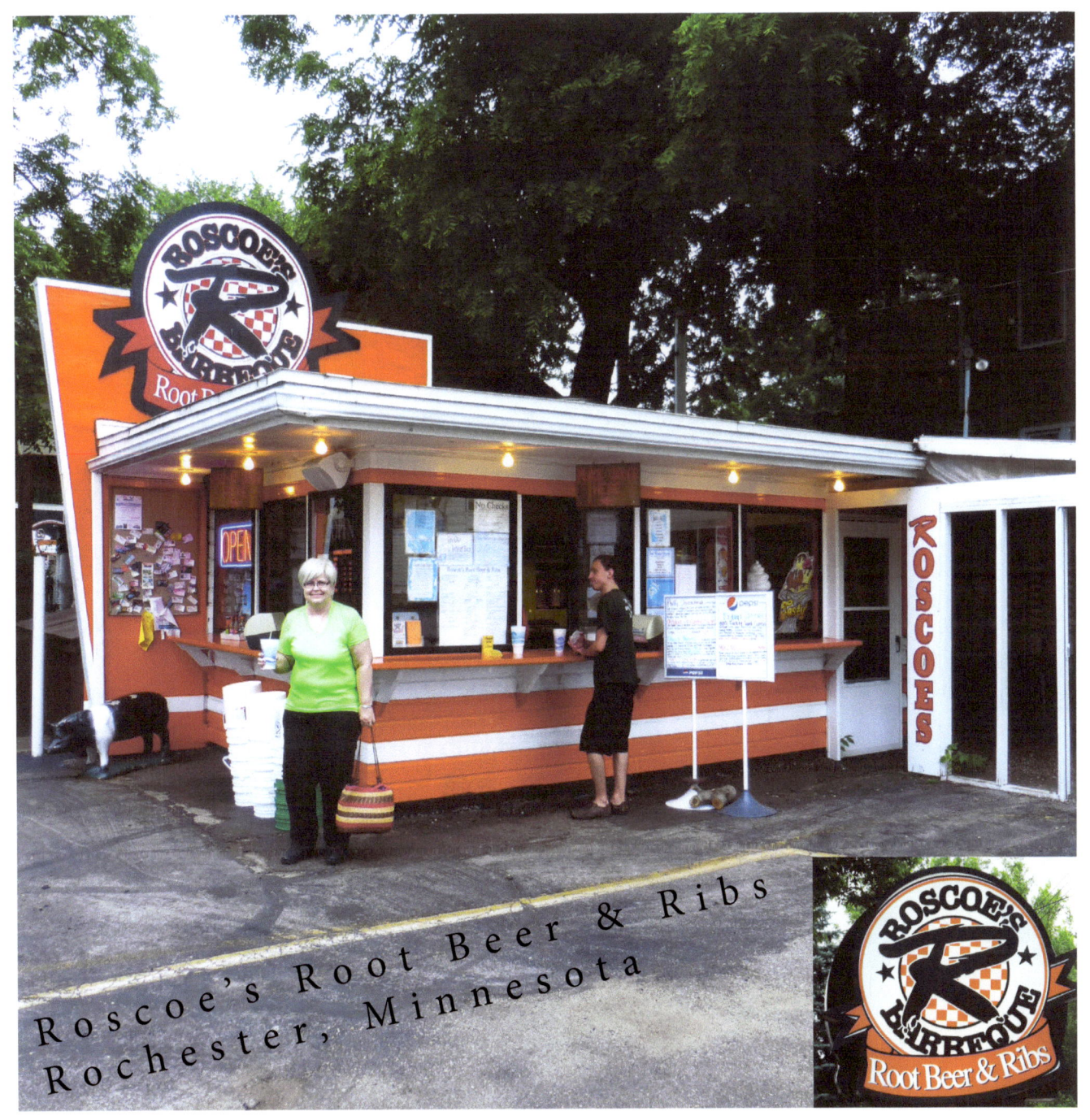

Roscoe's Root Beer & Ribs
Rochester, Minnesota

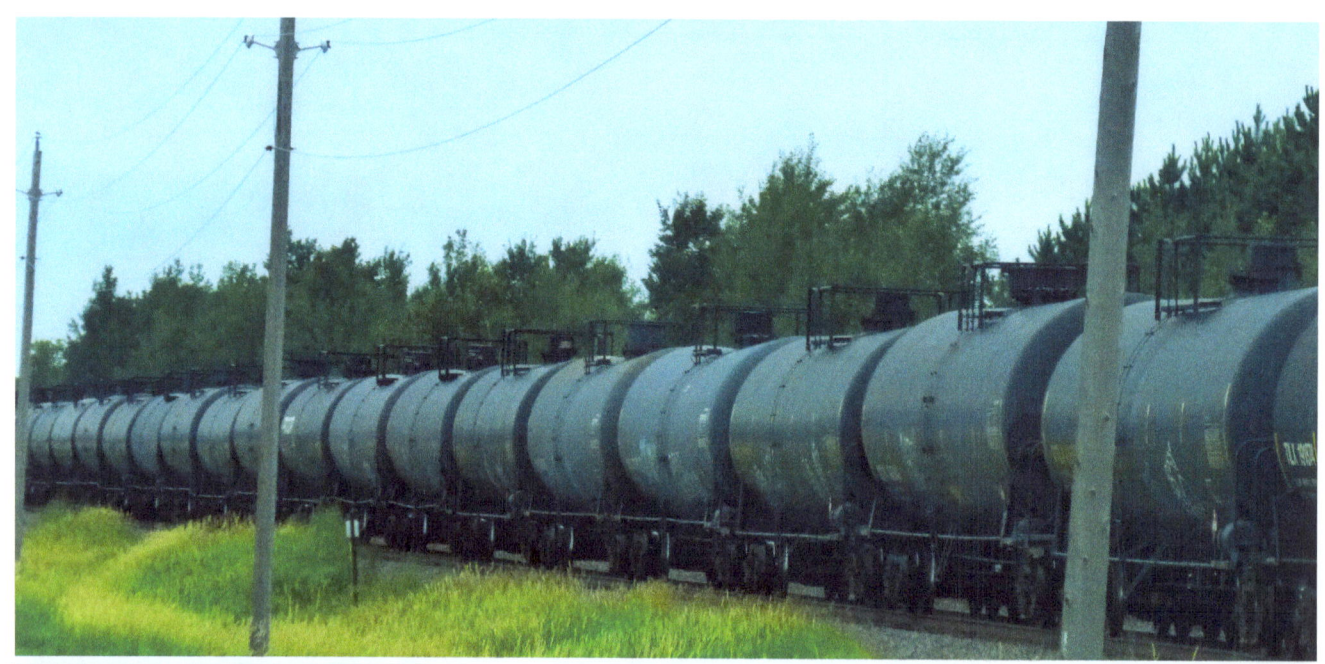

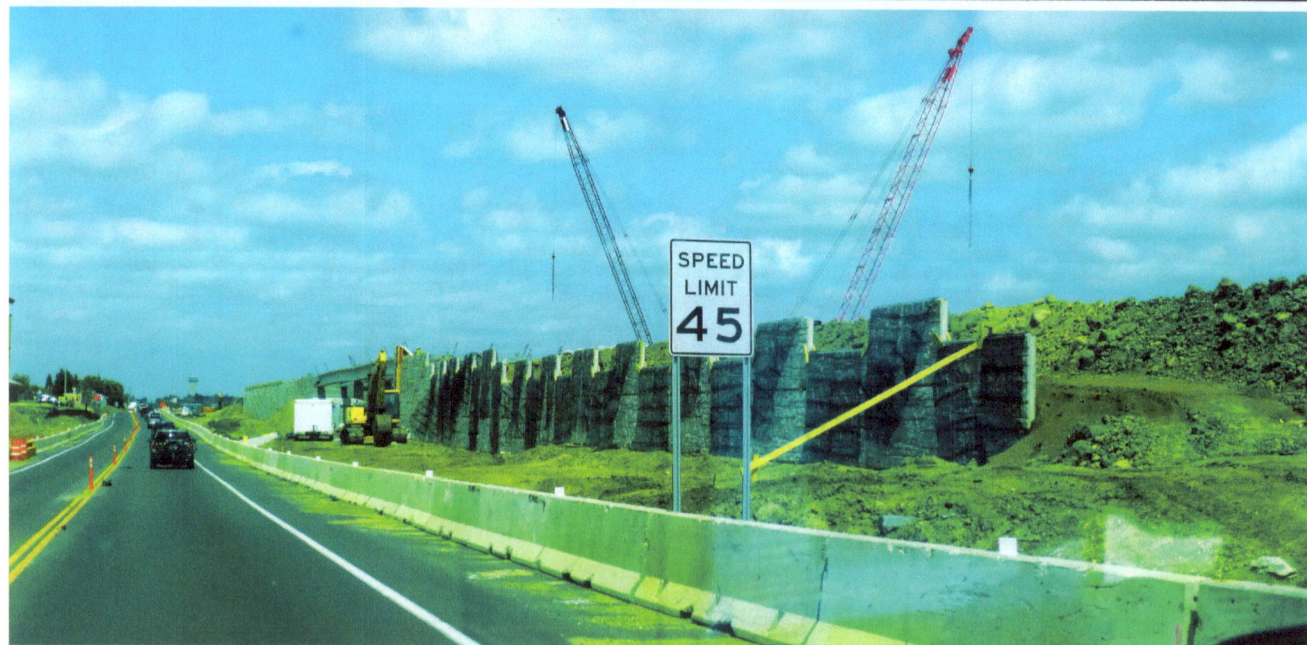

Road Construction & Trains in Central Minnesota

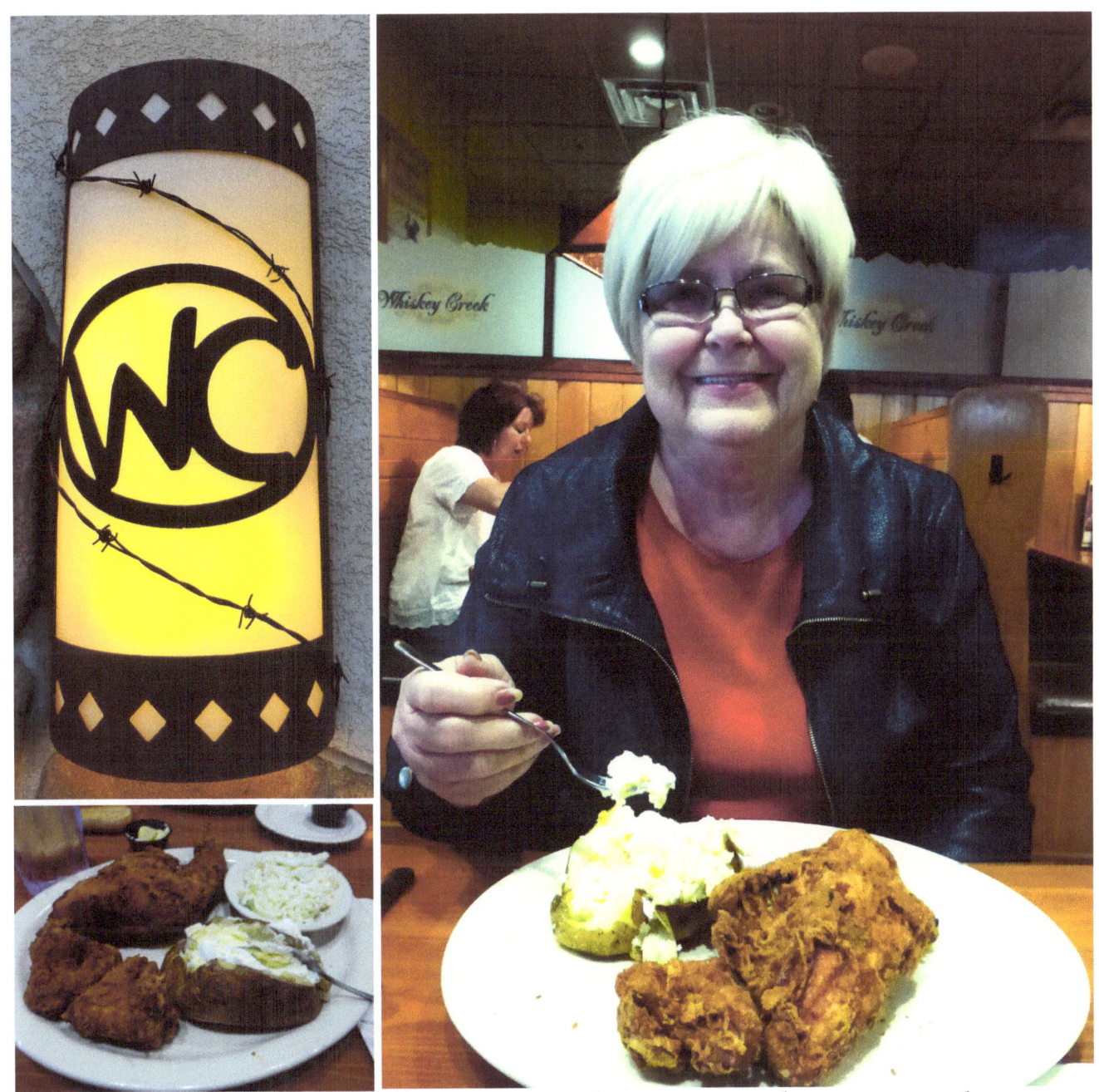

Broasted Chicken at Whiskey Creek in Rochester

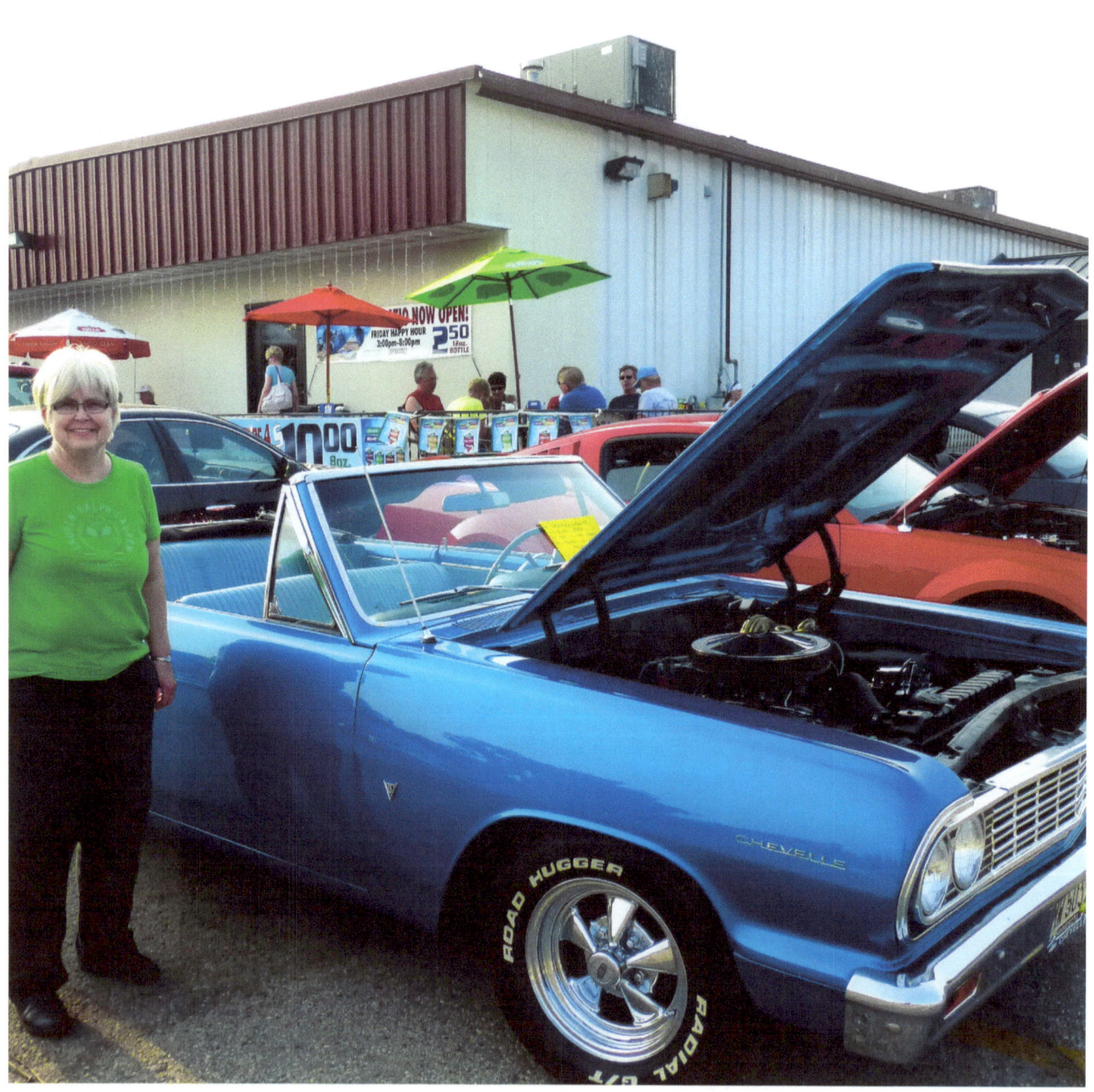

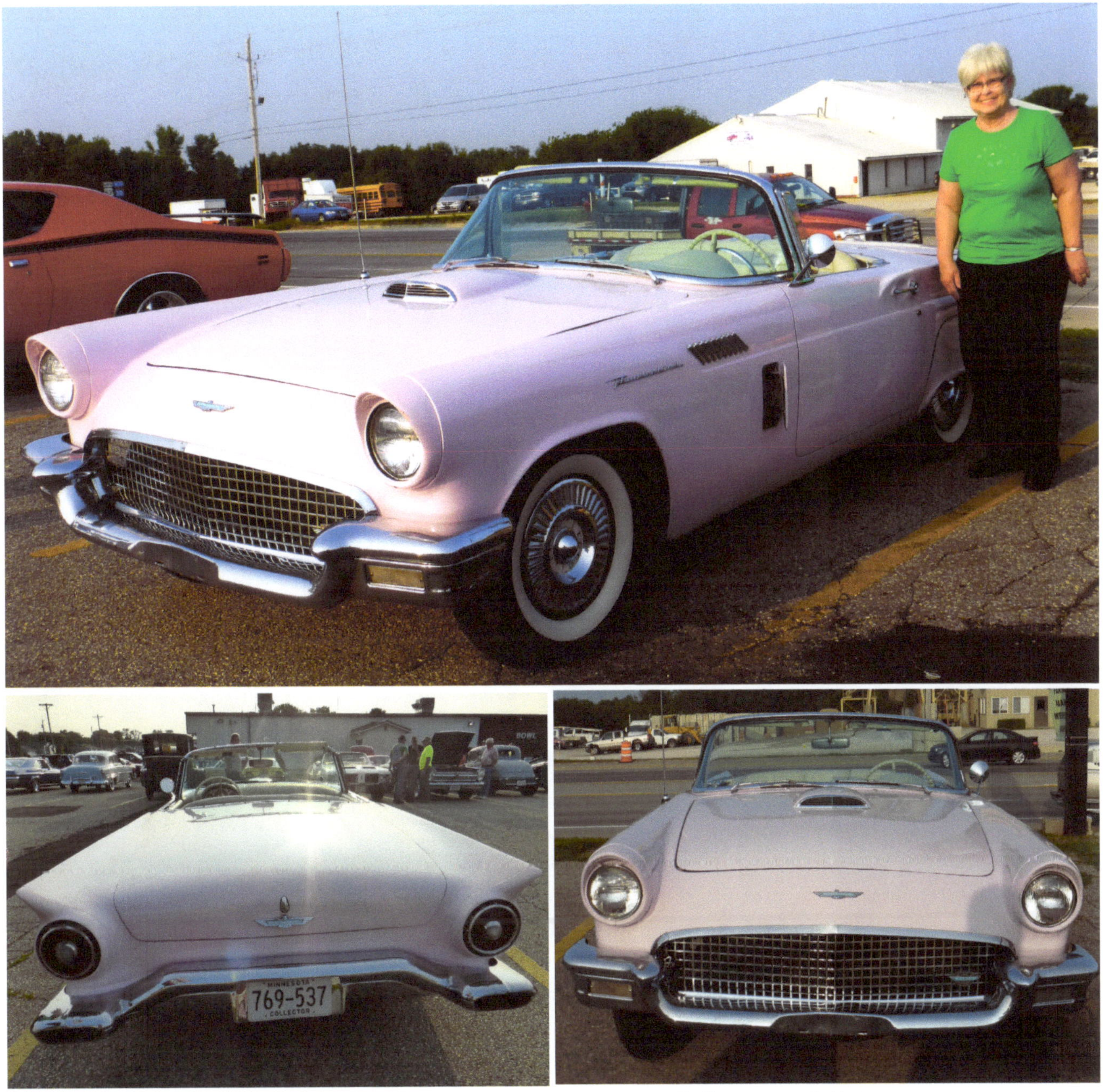

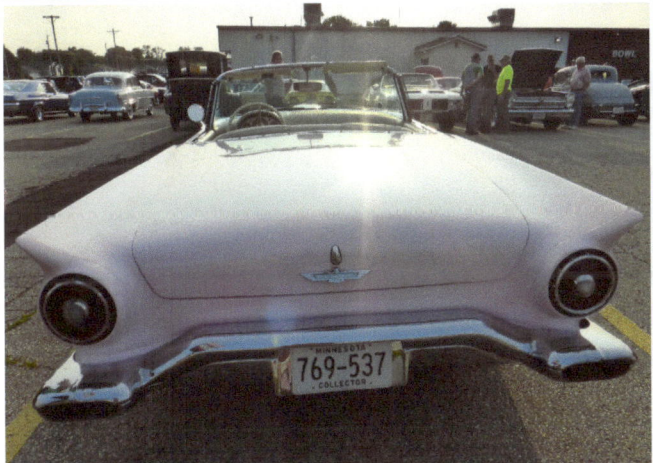

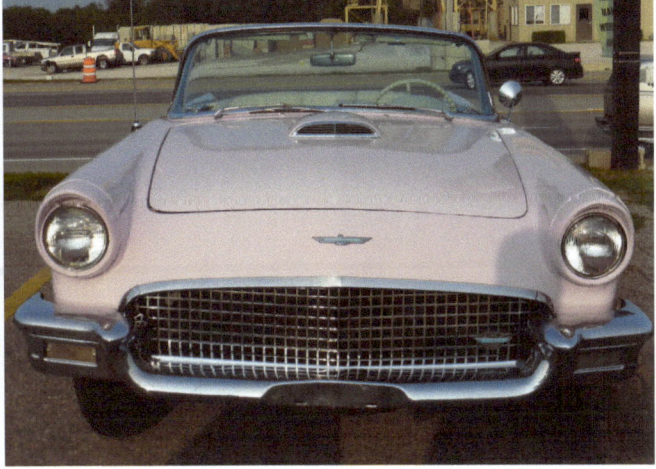

Car Show in Stewartville, Minnesota

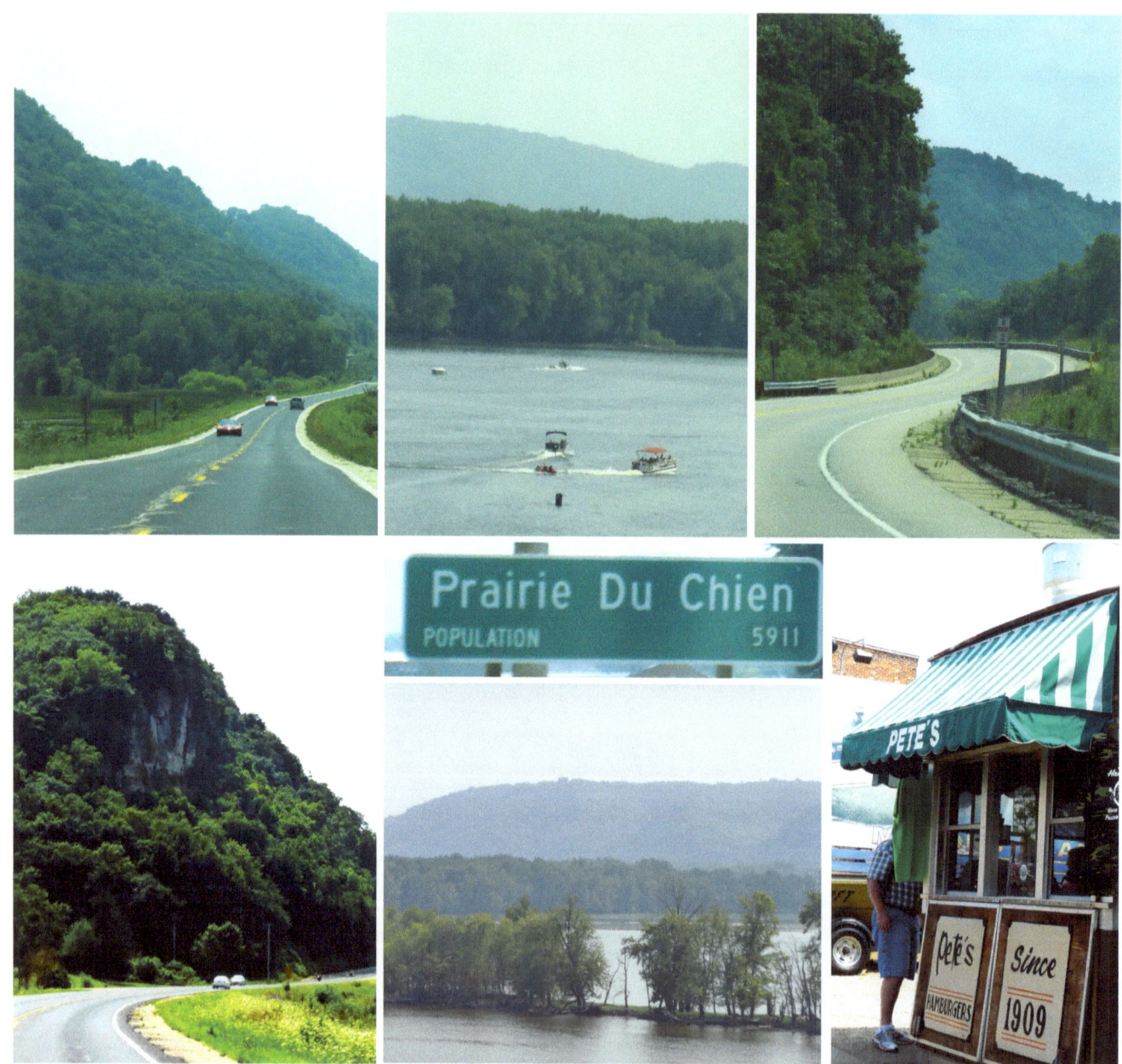

Driving Along Mississippi River Bluffs to
Prairie du Chien, Wisconsin

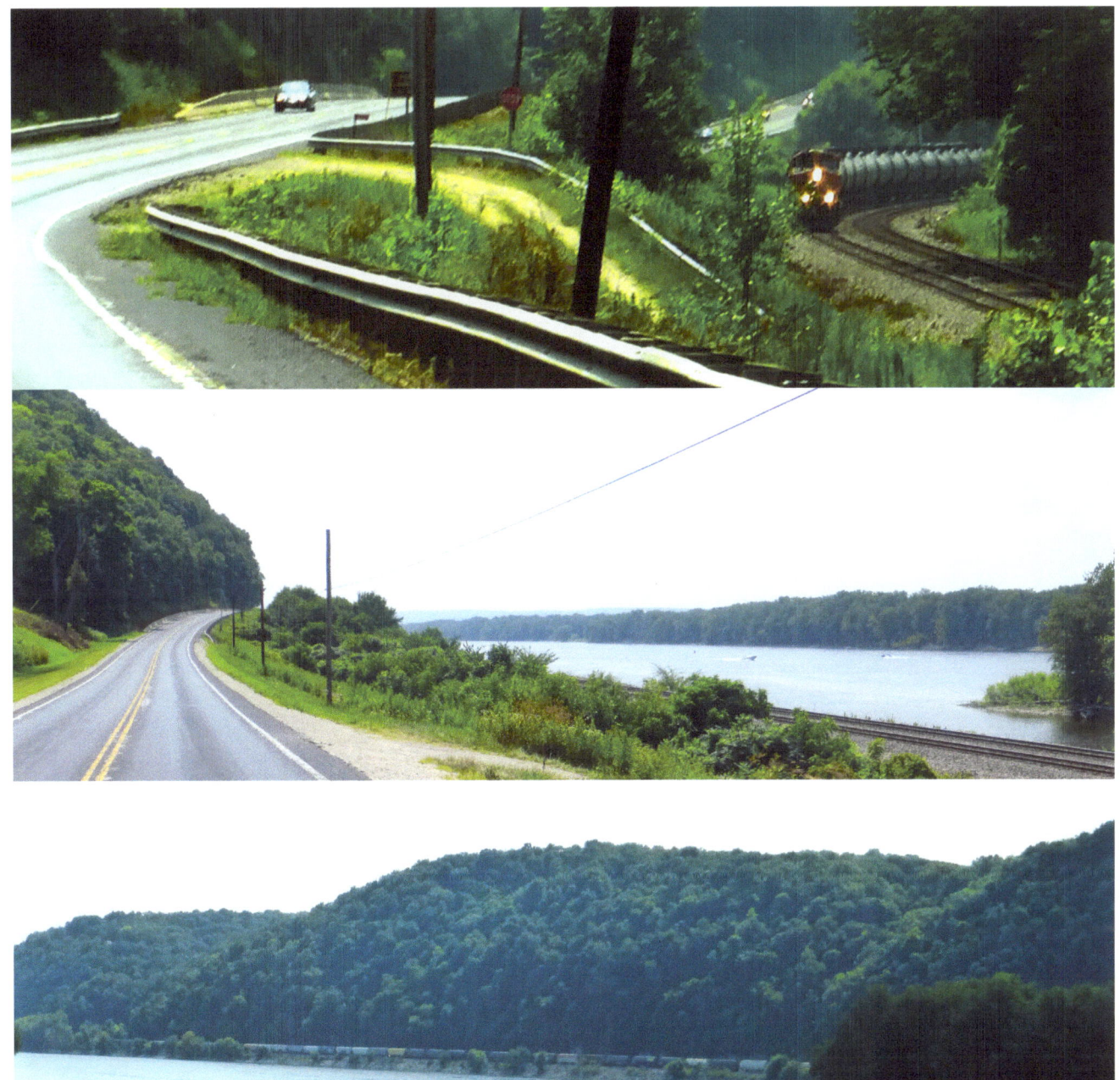

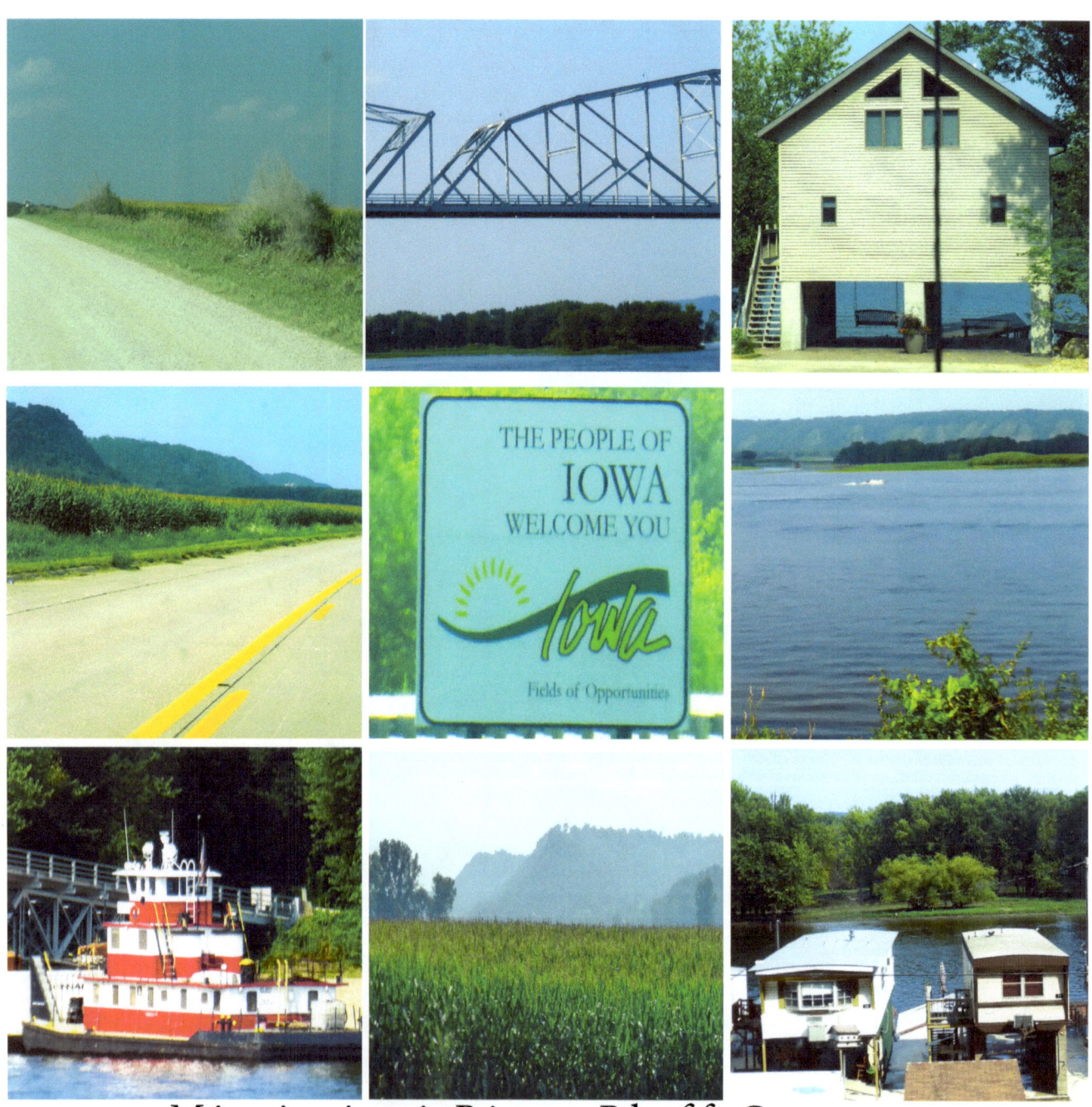

Mississippi River Bluff Country

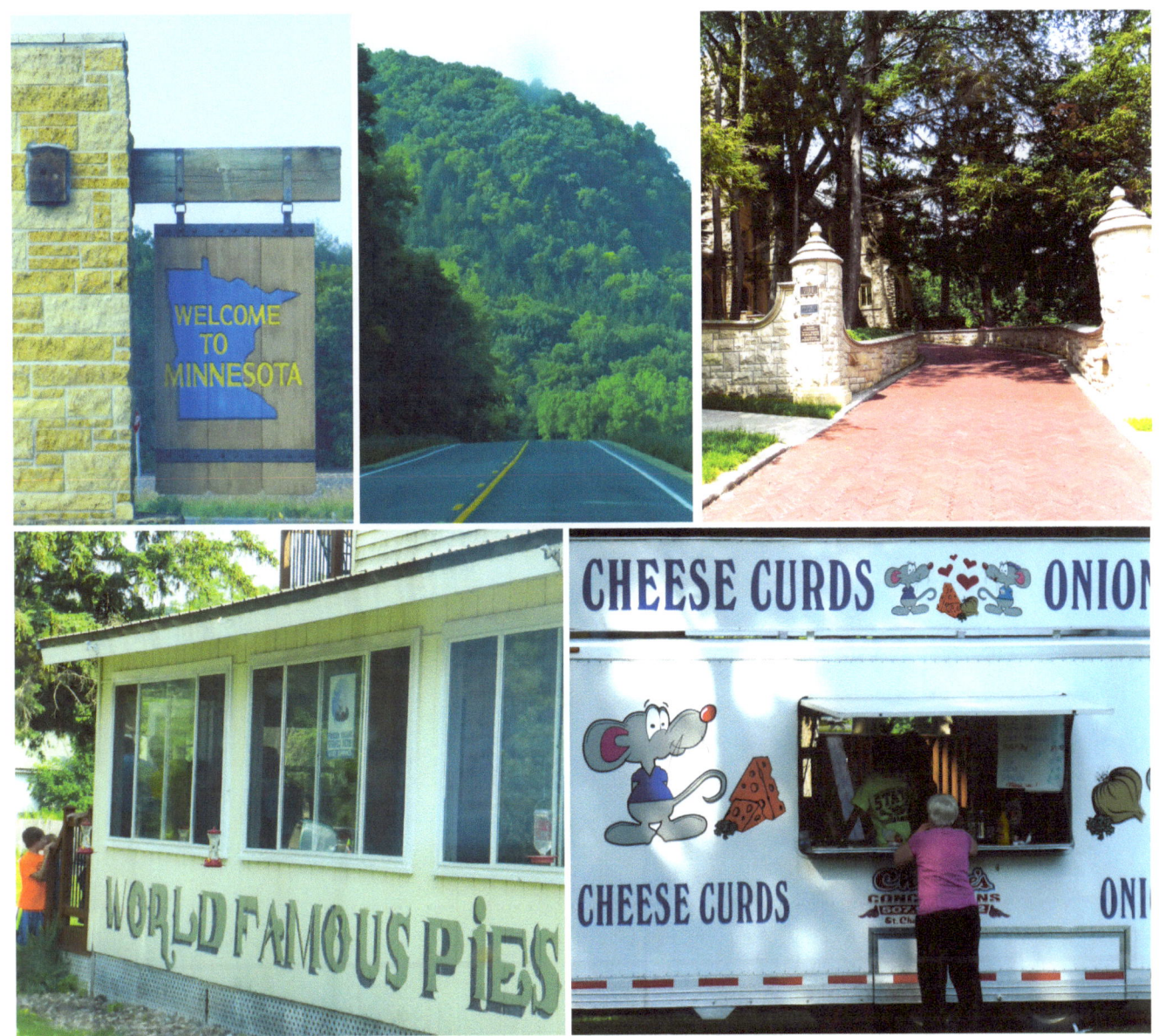

Dr. William J. Mayo House / Mayo Foundation House
Buffalo Bill Days in Lanesboro, MN
Aroma Pie Shop in Whalen, MN

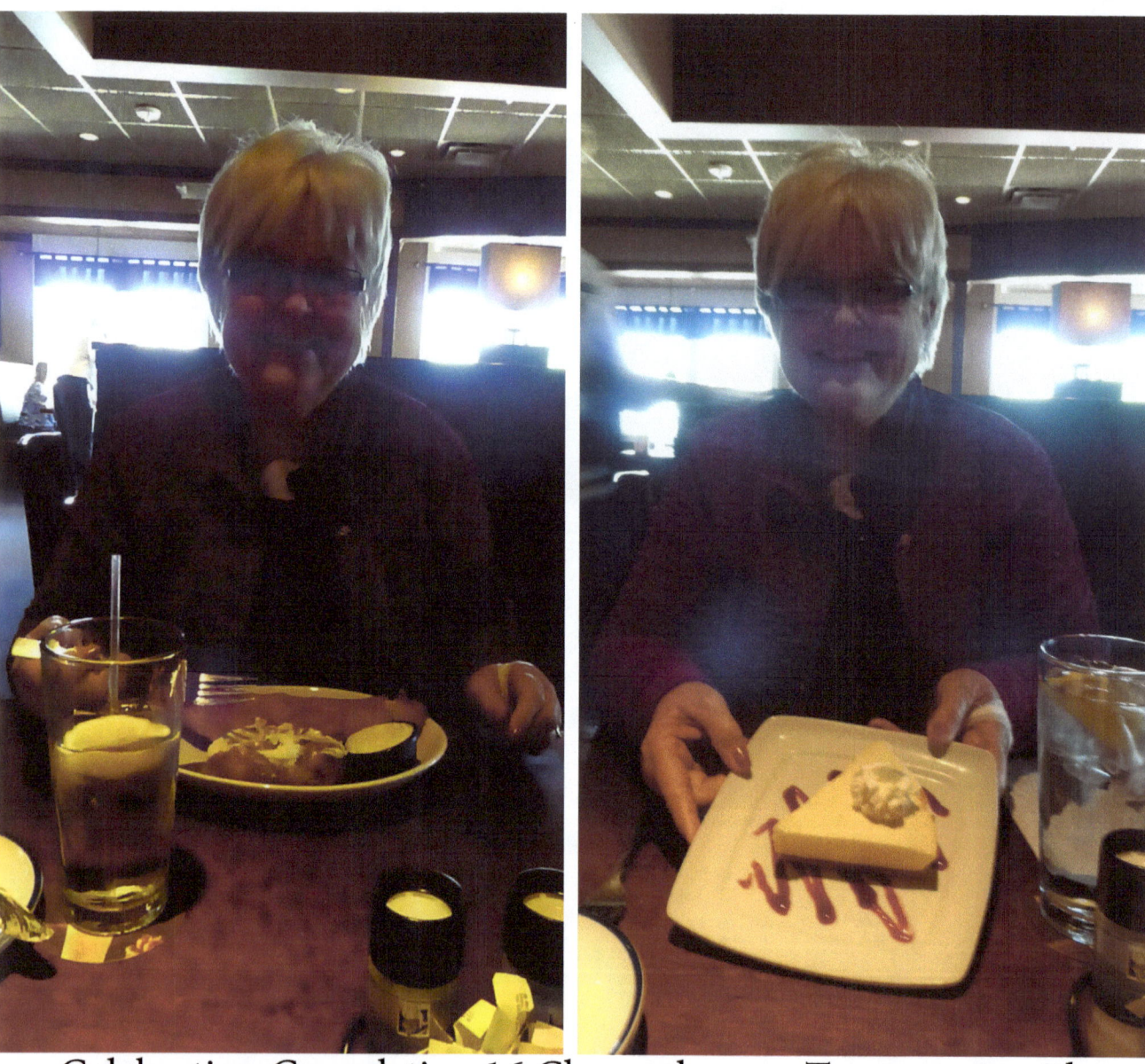

Celebrating Completing 16 Chemotherapy Treatments with Canadian Walleye at the Red Lobster. The Manager Brought Out Complimentary Cheesecake as a way to say Congratulations.

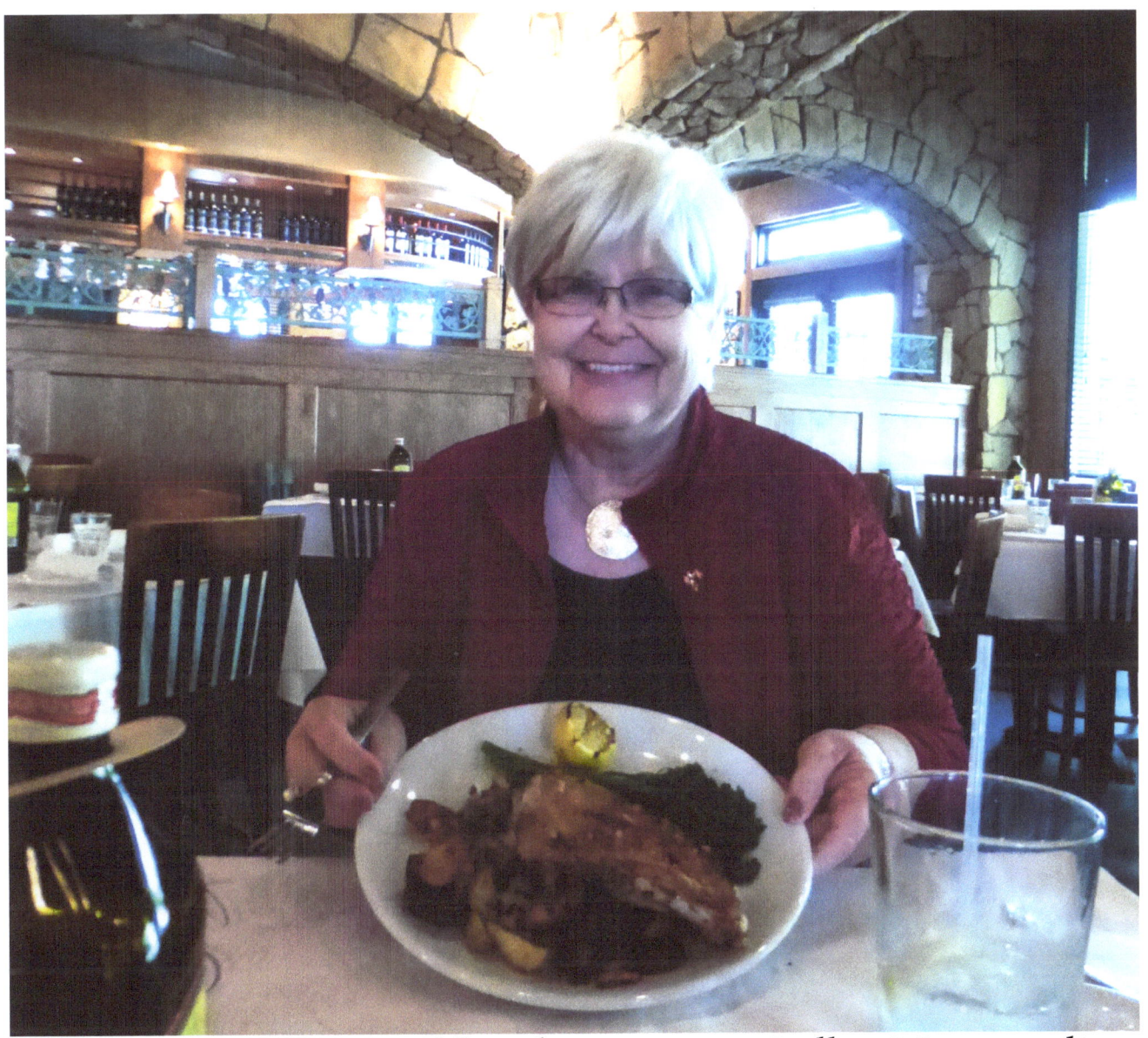

"Chicken Under A Brick" at the Macaroni Grill in Minneapolis.
Sage Roasted Chicken, Broccolini (Asparagus/Broccoli Cross), &
Garlic Rosemary Potatoes.

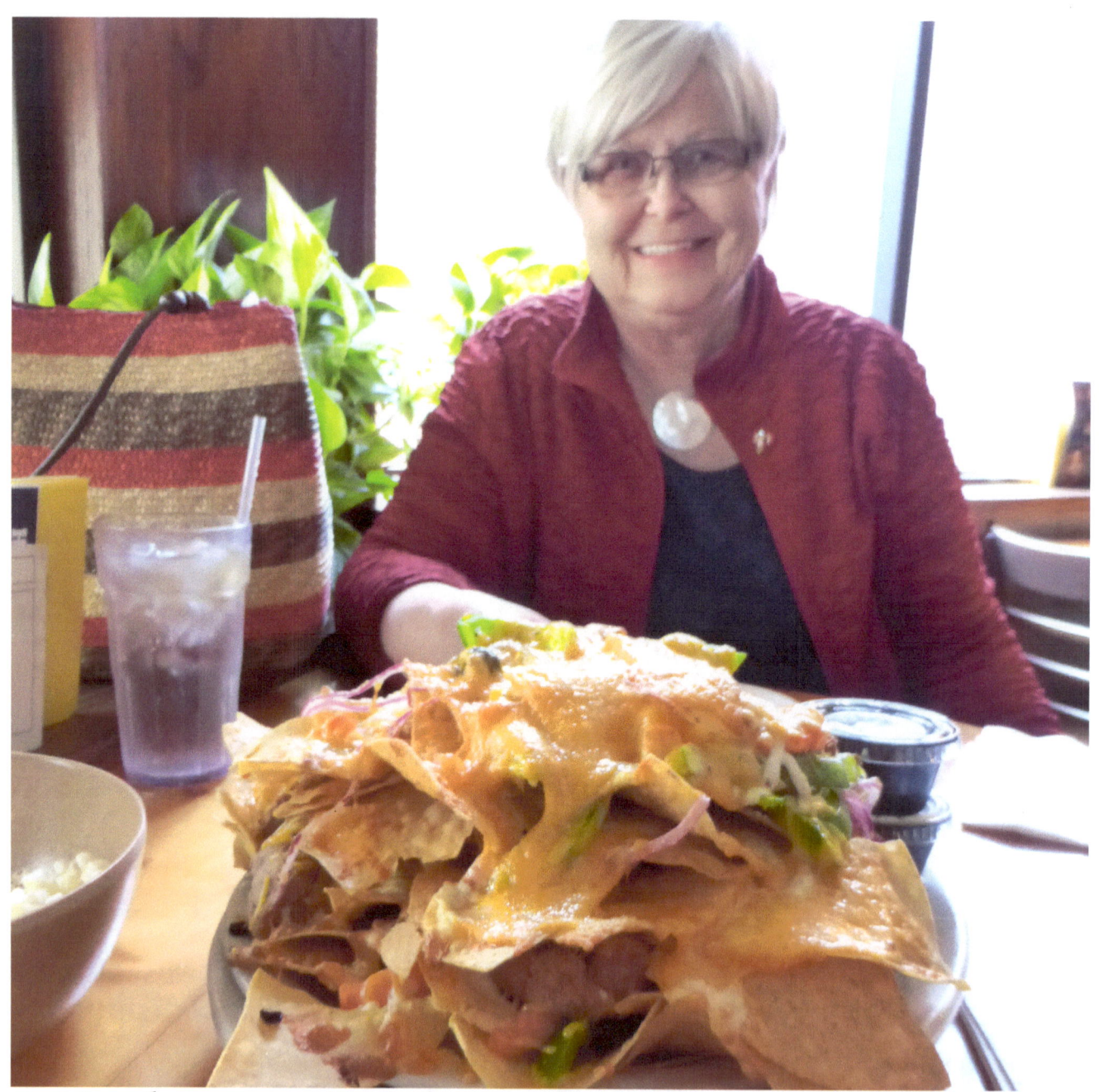

Nachos at Newt's in Downtown Rochester

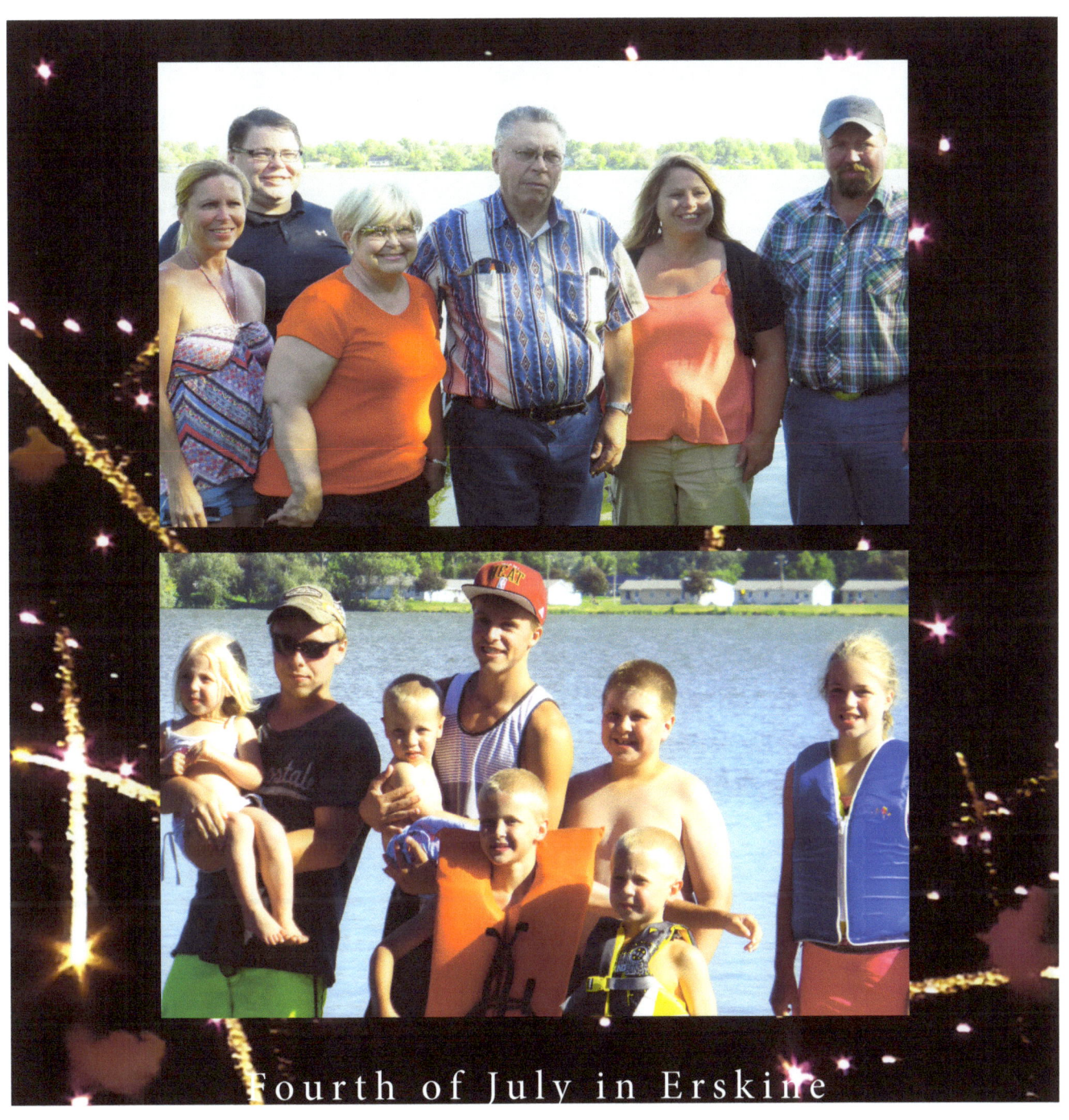

Fourth of July in Erskine

Zumbrota Covered Bridge
Minnesota's Last Covered Bridge

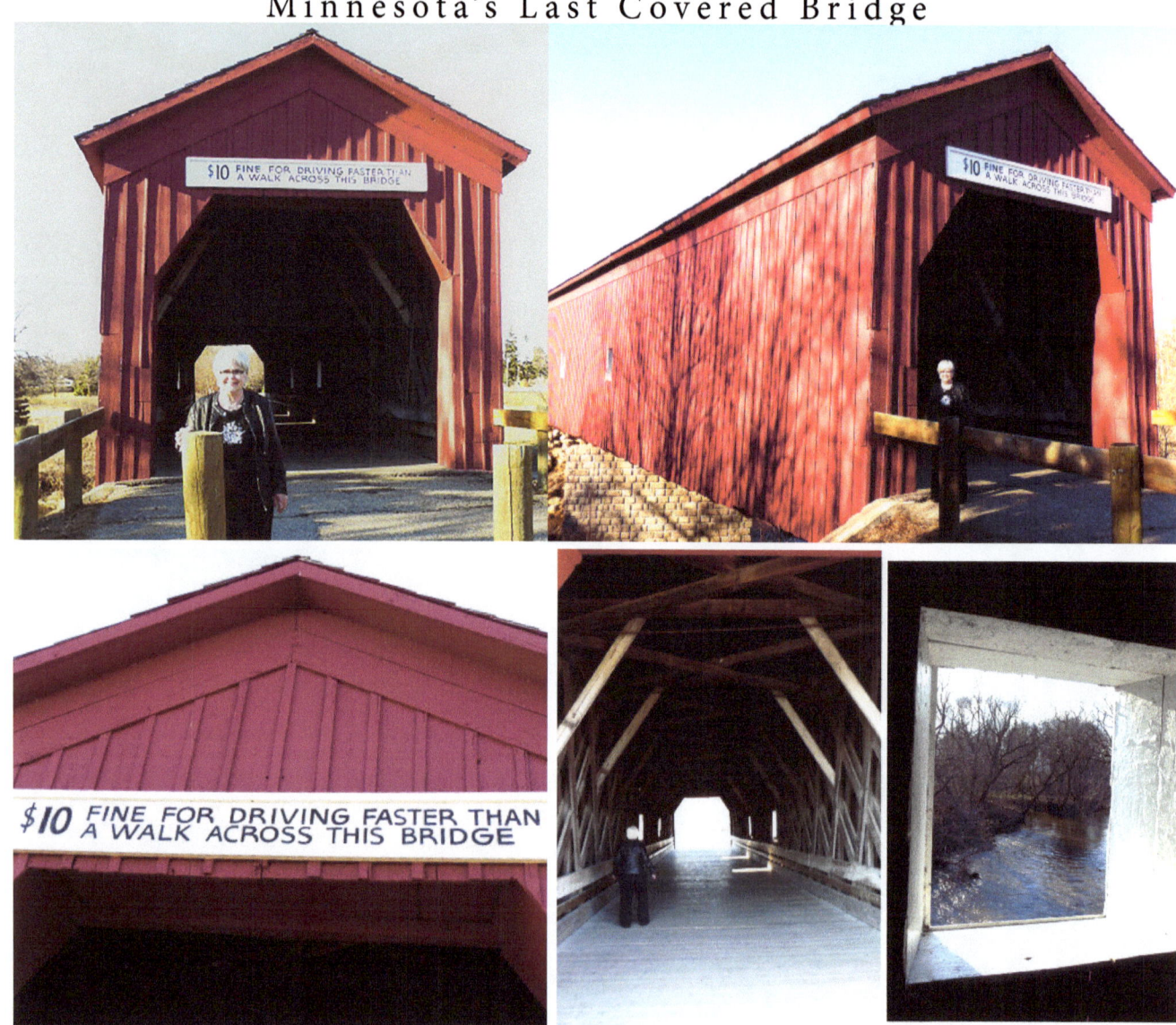

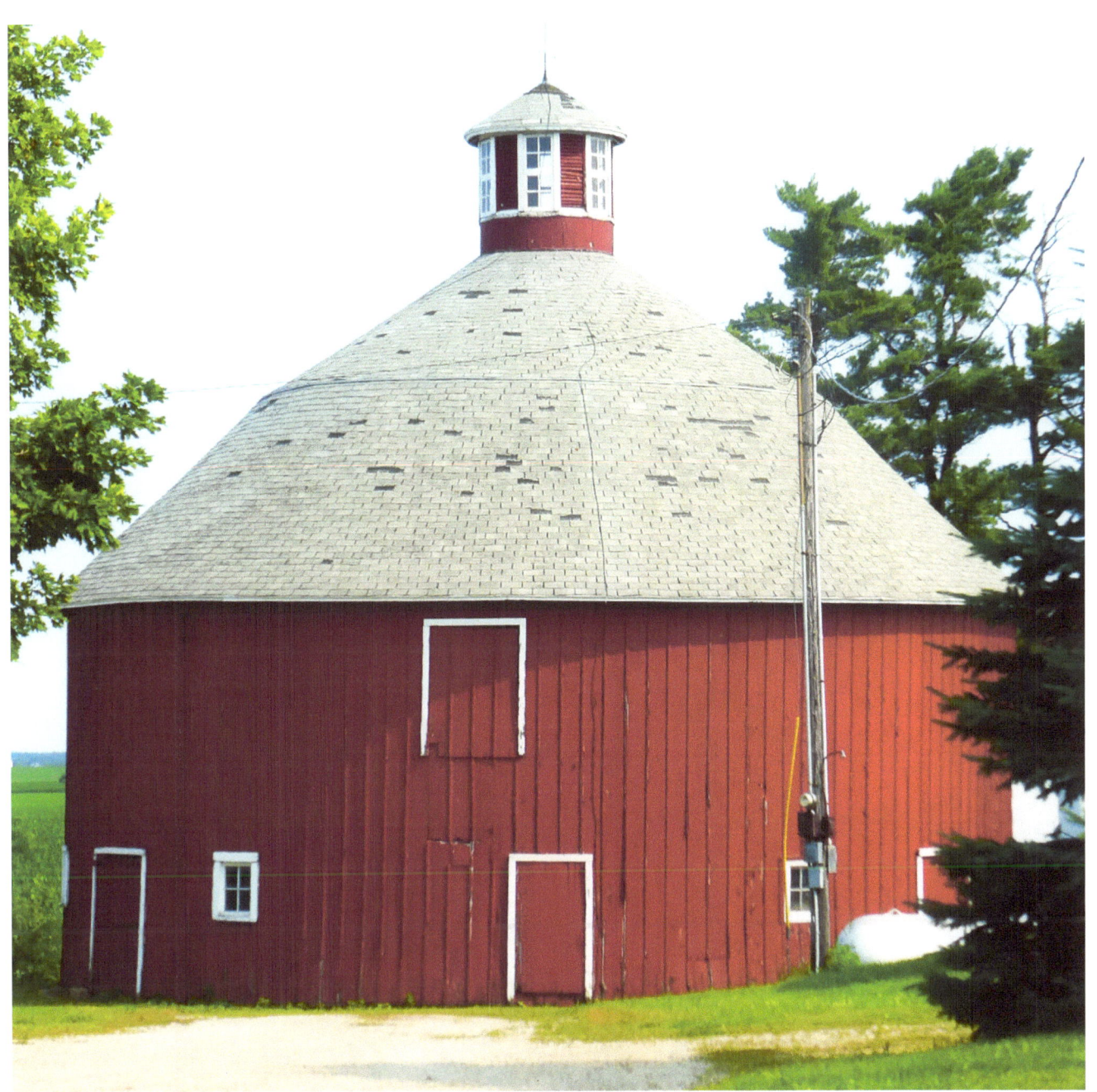

Round Barn

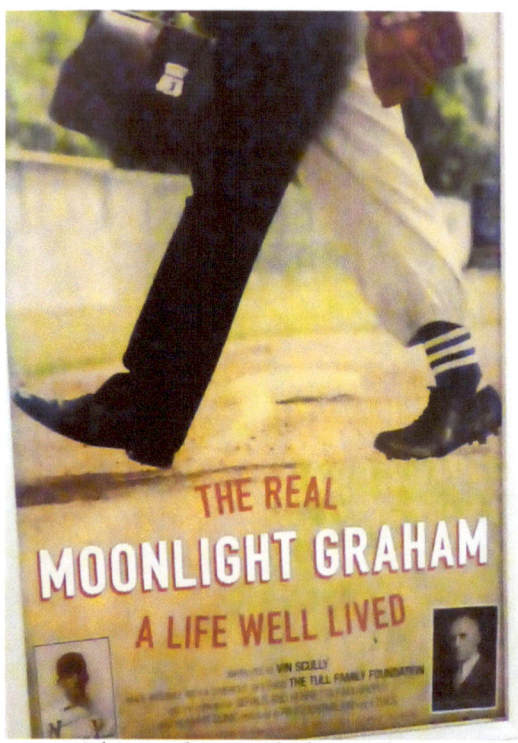

The Real Moonlight Graham:
A Life Well Lived
Mayo Clinic Doctor/Field of Dreams
Documentary Shown in the Subway
Level Auditorium of Gonda Building.

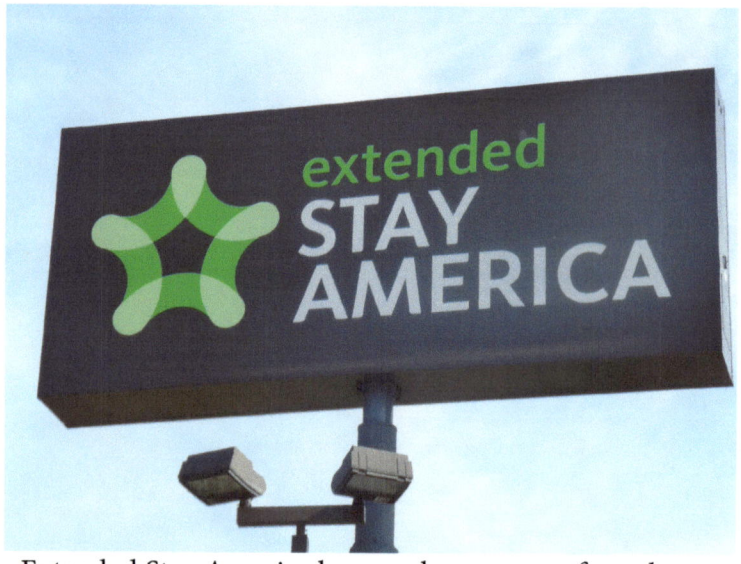

Extended Stay America became home-away-from-home when staying away from home, before staying at the Hope Lodge as the trade-off value of the rooms were the best fit for the budget. Each room comes with a small kitchen and fridge, making it possible to cook meals.

Trains are a common sight when driving between northern and southern Minnesota. Most trains are at least one-hundred train cars long, carrying oil from North Dakota oil fields.

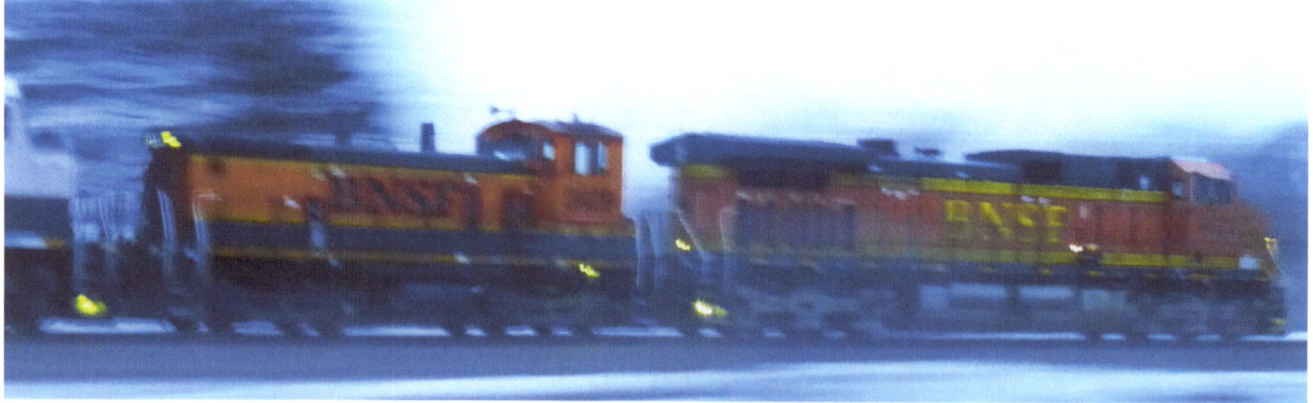

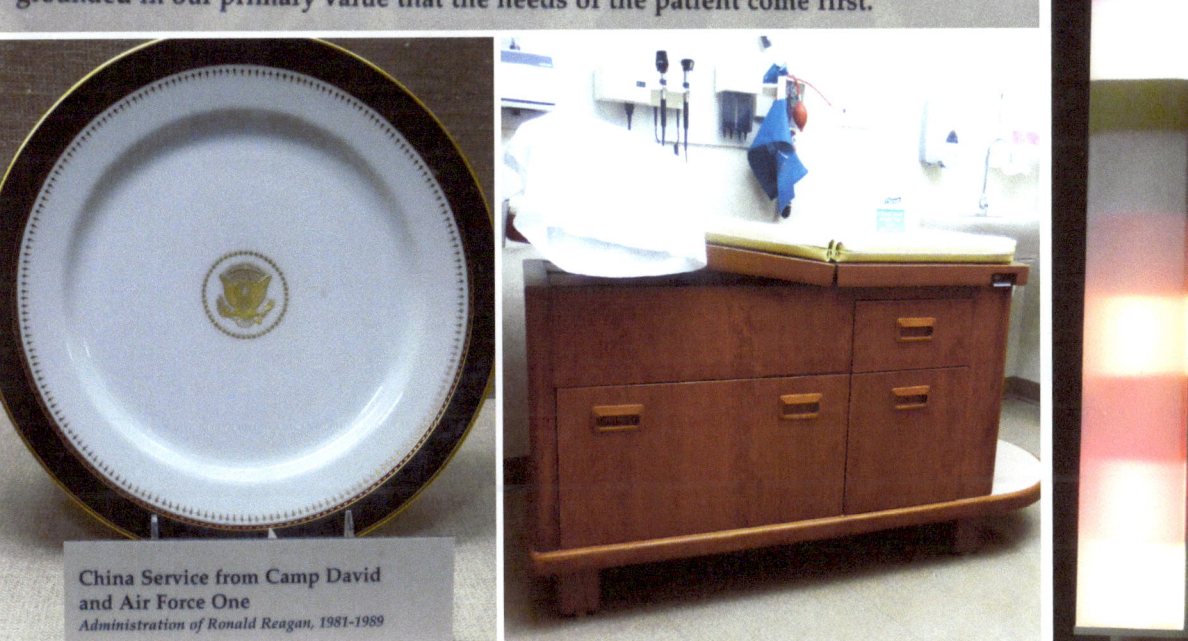

White House China
ICONS OF THE AMERICAN PRESIDENCY

Loaned from the Collection of Richard Townsend

The diverse patterns of White House china are enduring symbols of the American presidency. Designs evoke not only the personal tastes of First Families but also the great events of their administrations. Mayo Clinic expresses appreciation to Mr. Townsend for generously loaning selections from his acclaimed collection.

Mayo Clinic has an unparalleled relationship with presidential and vice presidential families—spanning generations and administrations from Abraham Lincoln to the present. This relationship is nonpartisan and nonpolitical. It is grounded in our primary value that the needs of the patient come first.

China Service from Camp David and Air Force One
Administration of Ronald Reagan, 1981-1989

309

White House China | Mayo Clinic Exam Table
Light Outside of Exam Room When a Doctor is With a Patient.

Mayo Clinic Art

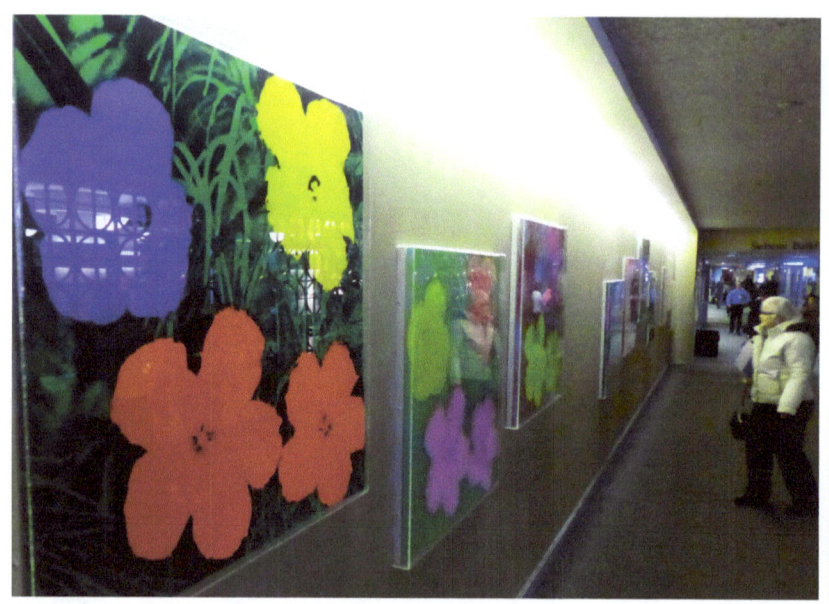

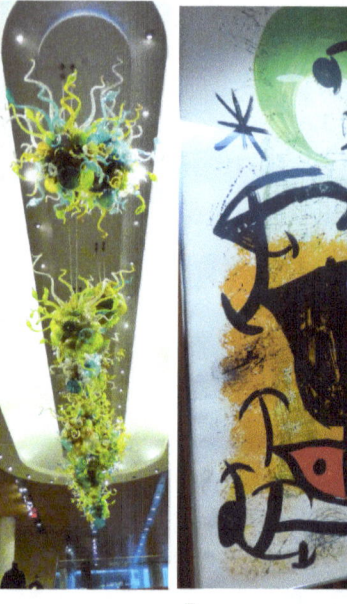

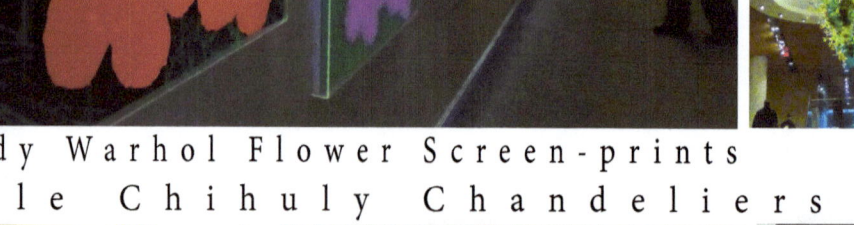

Andy Warhol Flower Screen-prints
Dale Chihuly Chandeliers

Joan Miro
Lithograph

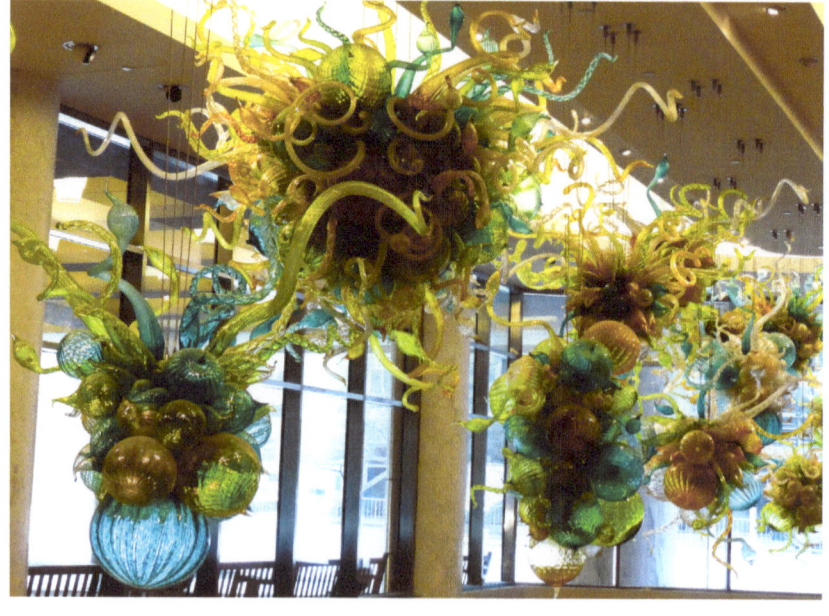

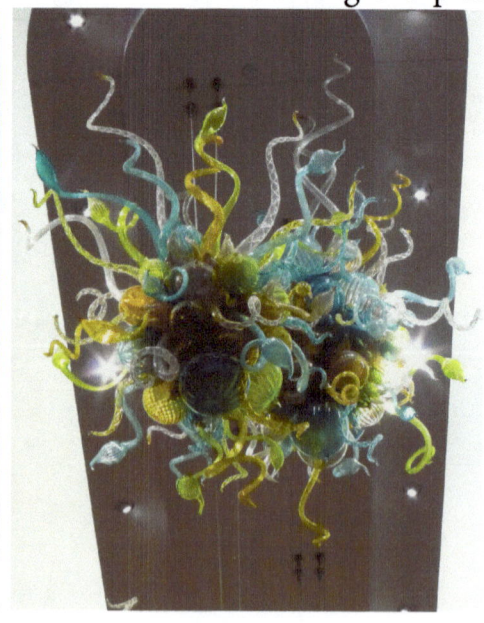

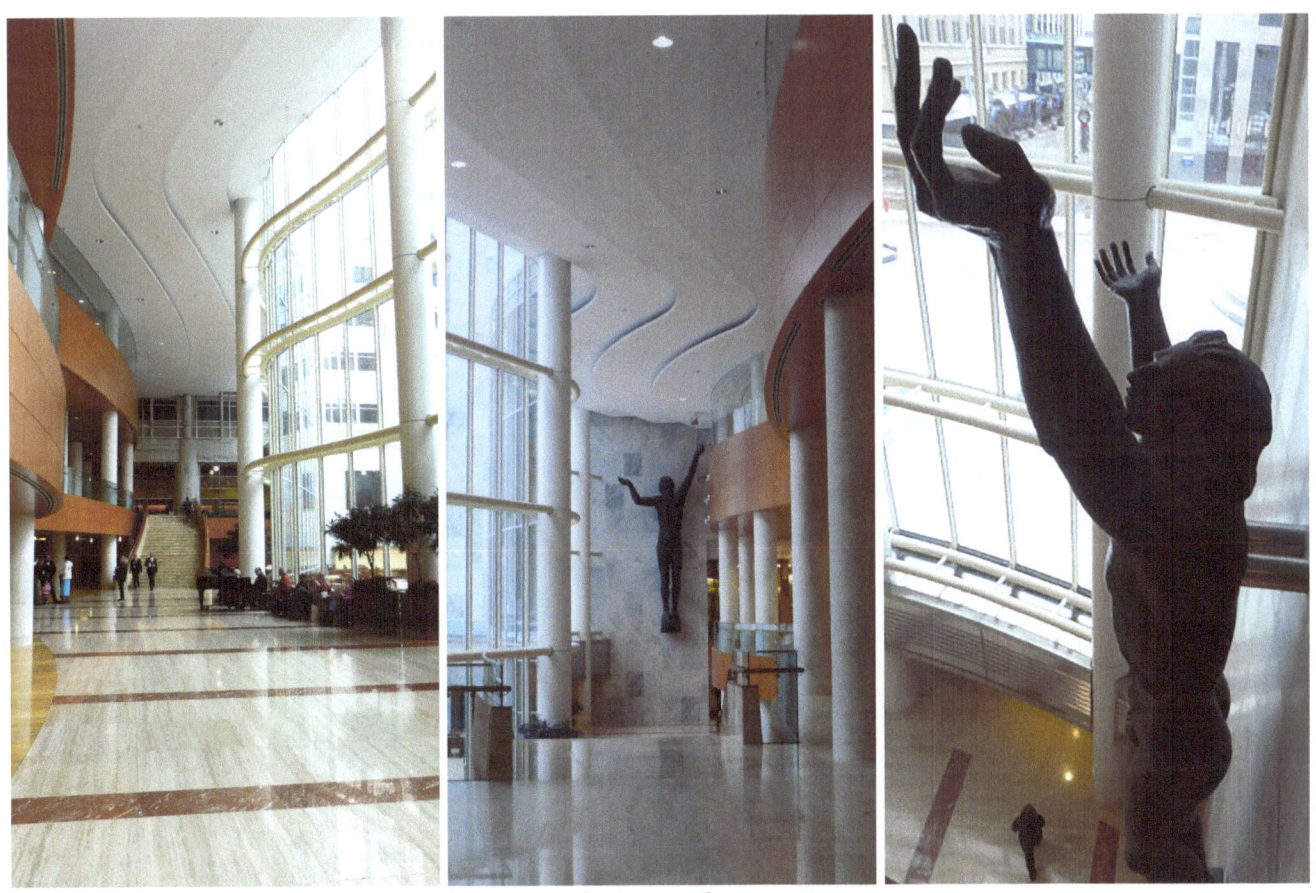

Man and Freedom Statue

"Soaring above the Nathan Landrum Atrium inside the Gonda Building is the Man and Freedom Statue created by Yugoslavian sculptor Ivan Mestrovic in 1954, at his studio on the Notre Dame University campus in Indiana. A peasant sheepherder, born in Croatia in 1883, he managed to study at the Vienna Academy of Fine Arts and work in Rome before his family came to America."

"Mestrovic meant this work to celebrate symbolically the Croation/Serbian overthrow of domination by the Austro-Hungarian empire. Mestrovic explained his work by saying: "To all living beings ... individual freedom is the most precious, free not only physically but spiritually as well." As a patient walks across the atrium expanse, viewing the 28-foot, 6,900-pound cast bronze sculpture with hands outstretched towards the heavens, one's spirits are lifted, no matter how burdensome one's own illness might be."

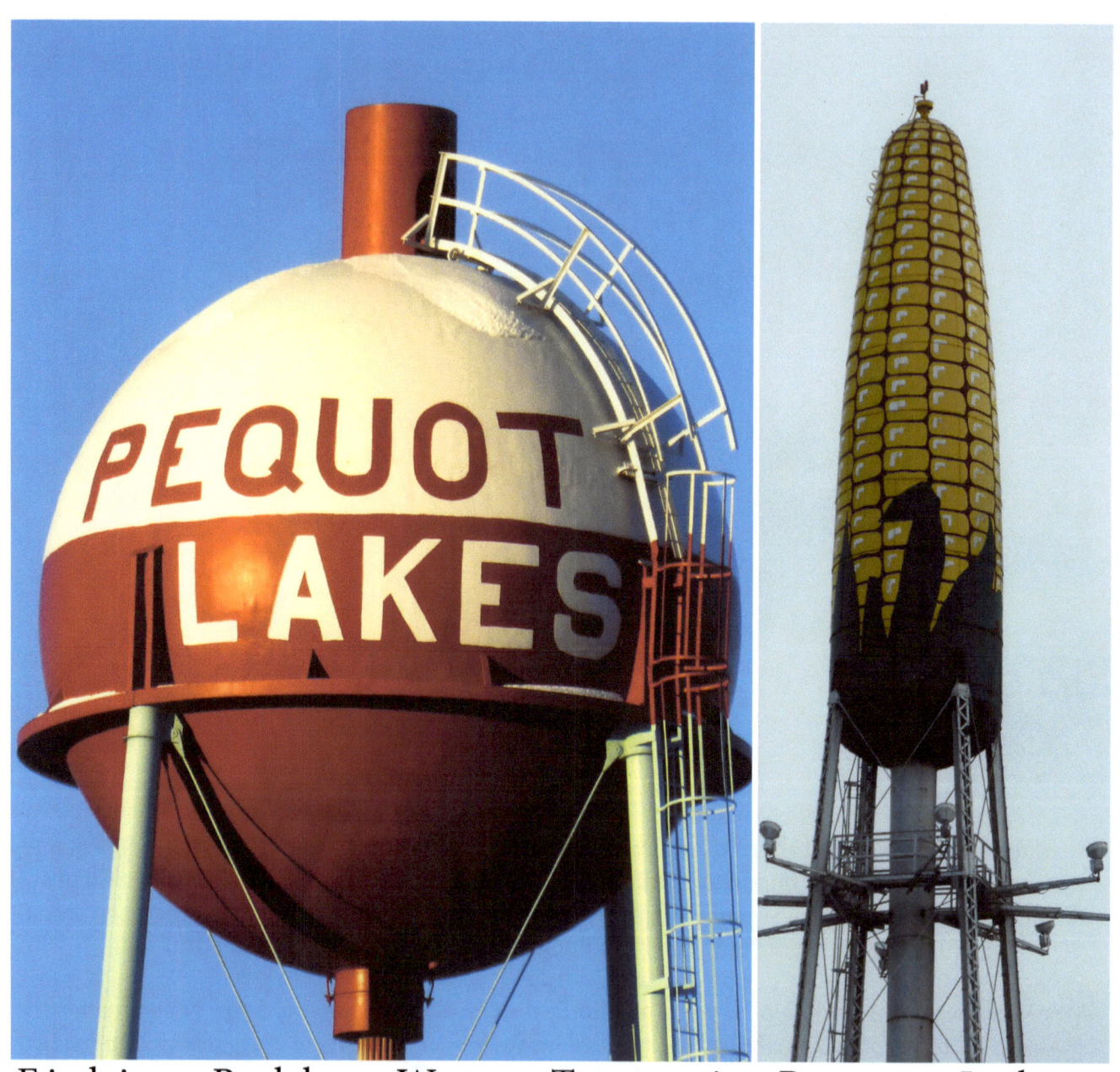

Fishing Bobber Water Tower in Pequot Lakes.
Corn Cob Water Tower in Rochester.

Paul Bunyan
"A Symbol of Bigness, Strength, and Vitality."

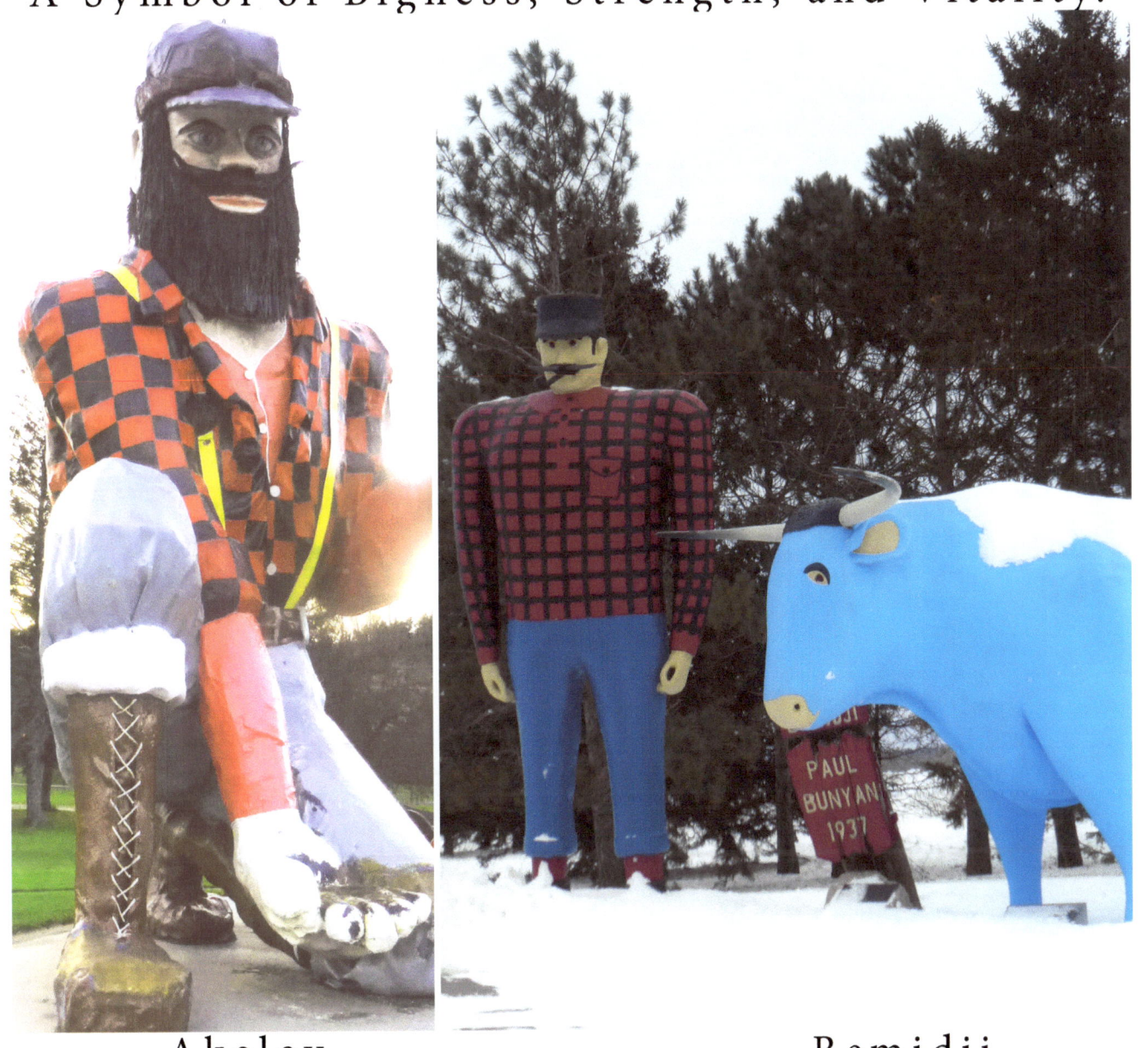

Akeley   Bemidji

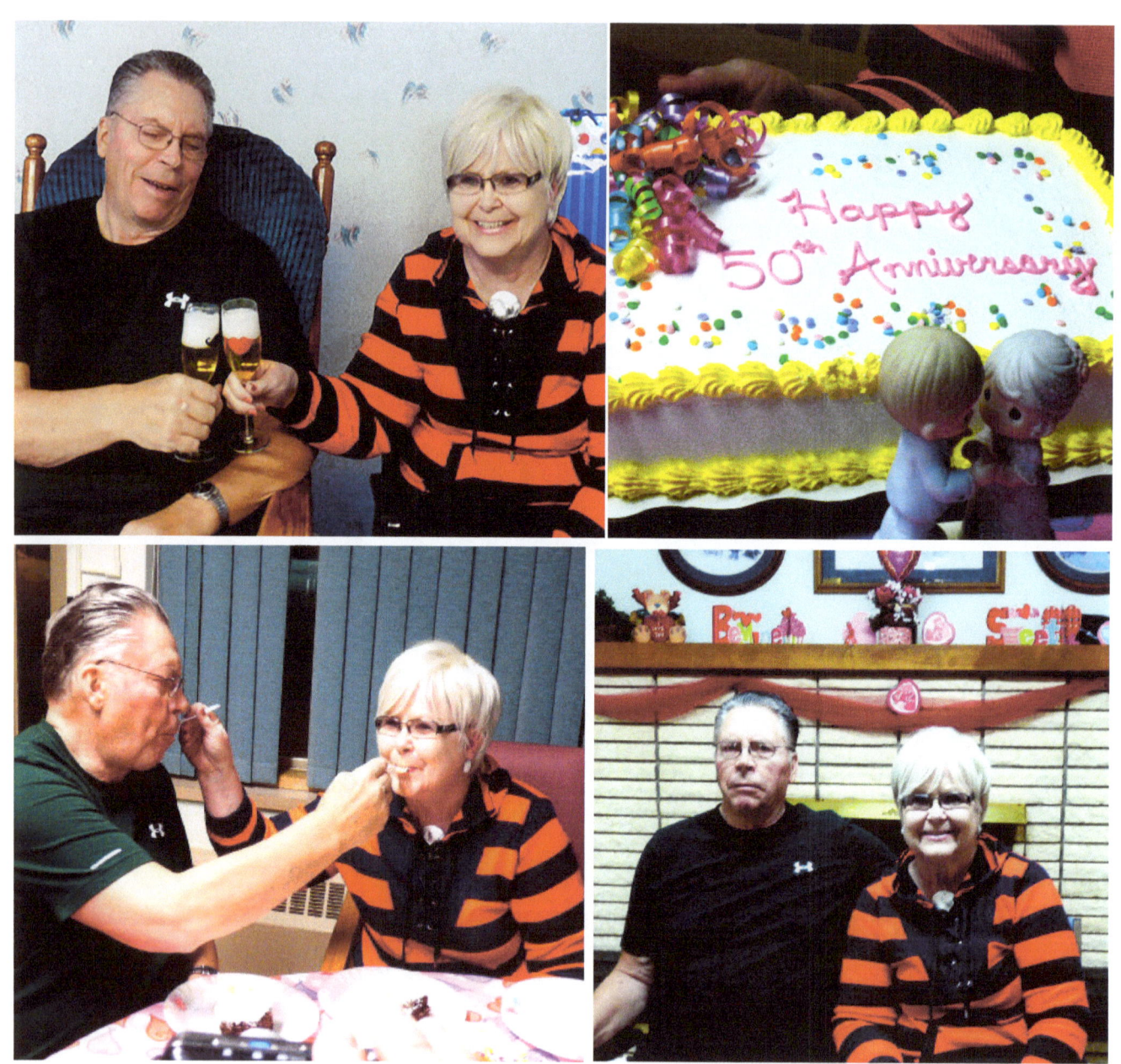

50TH Wedding Anniversary
February 15, 2014

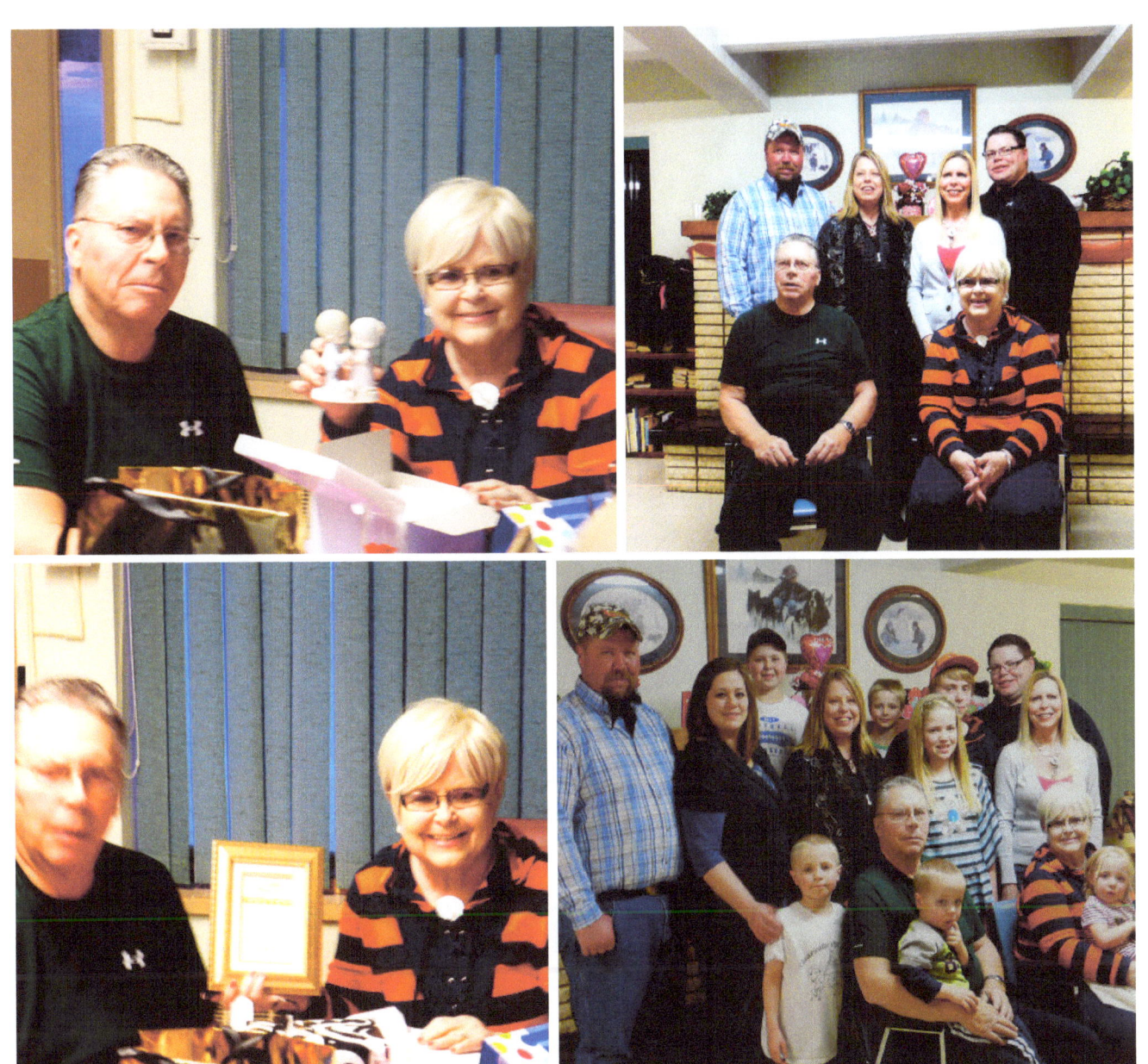

50TH Wedding Anniversary
February 15, 2014

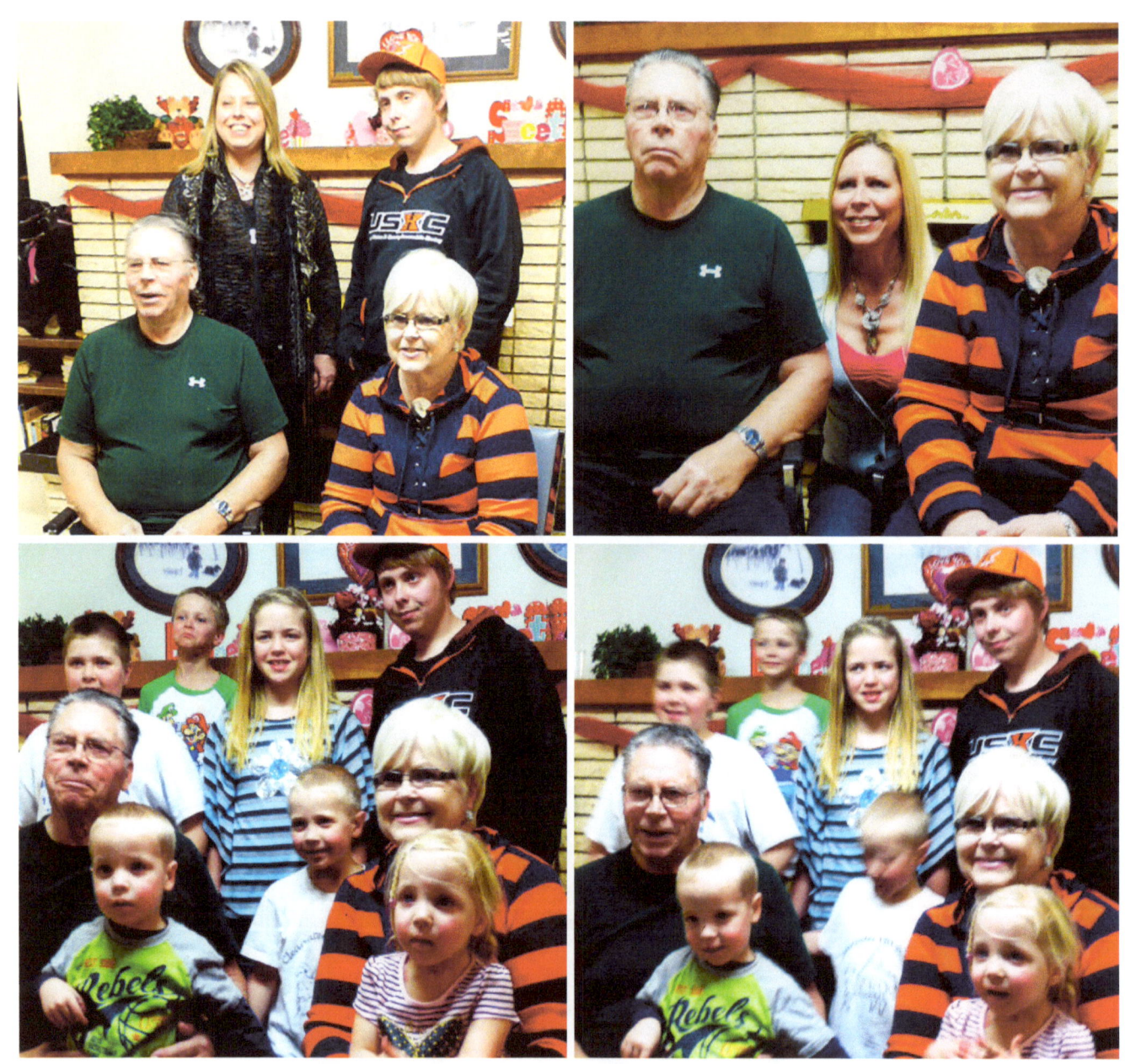

50TH Wedding Anniversary
February 15, 2014

Date: May 3, 2014   **Time: 4:30-8:30 PM**

Location: Gully Hall

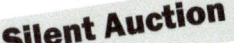

Howard & Linda Hanson Benefit

Silent Auction

Music by: "The Watnes"

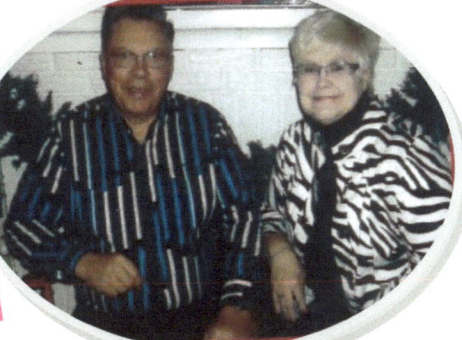

Bake Sale

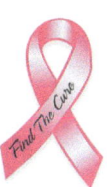

Meal Served from 4:30-8:00 PM - Free will offering

Roast Beef on Bun, Potato Salad, Beans, Chips, Pickles, Dessert

Linda was diagnosed last fall with stage 3-breast cancer. She has had three surgeries and is presently traveling each week for chemotherapy at the Mayo Clinic. Recently she was hospitalized with blood clots (pulmonary embolisms) in her lungs as a result of the cancers reaction to chemotherapy. Expensive medications are needed to prevent additional blood clots, from now until several months after completing all chemo/radiation treatments. Howard has been very ill these past 6 months. He has been hospitalized several times and was in a nursing home as a result of a bladder infection, blood clots in his lungs, etc. These conditions have enhanced the effects of his Parkinson's Disease.

The out-of-pocket expense for medications, clinic and hospital bills for Linda and Howard have become overwhelming. Any support would be greatly appreciated and will be used for medical expenses. Thank you!

Date: Sat, May 3, 2014

Time: 4:30-8:30 PM

Location: Hall @ Gully, MN

Dinner: 4:30-8:00 PM

Bake Sale: 4:30 PM til gone

Silent Auction: Ends @ 8:00 PM

Music: Provided by the Watne's

Donations are being taken for the Bake Sale & Silent Auction and can be dropped off @ the Hall in Gully the day of the benefit or contact:
Joanne-(218) 686-0489 **or**
Dean & Naomi-(218) 268-4555

If you are unable to attend and would like to contribute donations can be sent to:
Border State Bank
PO Box 599
1528 Hwy 59 South
Thief River Falls, MN 56701
Checks Payable to: Howard & Linda Hanson Benefit

Supplemental Funds provided by Pennington/Red Lake Counties Chapter of Thrivent Financial for Lutherans.

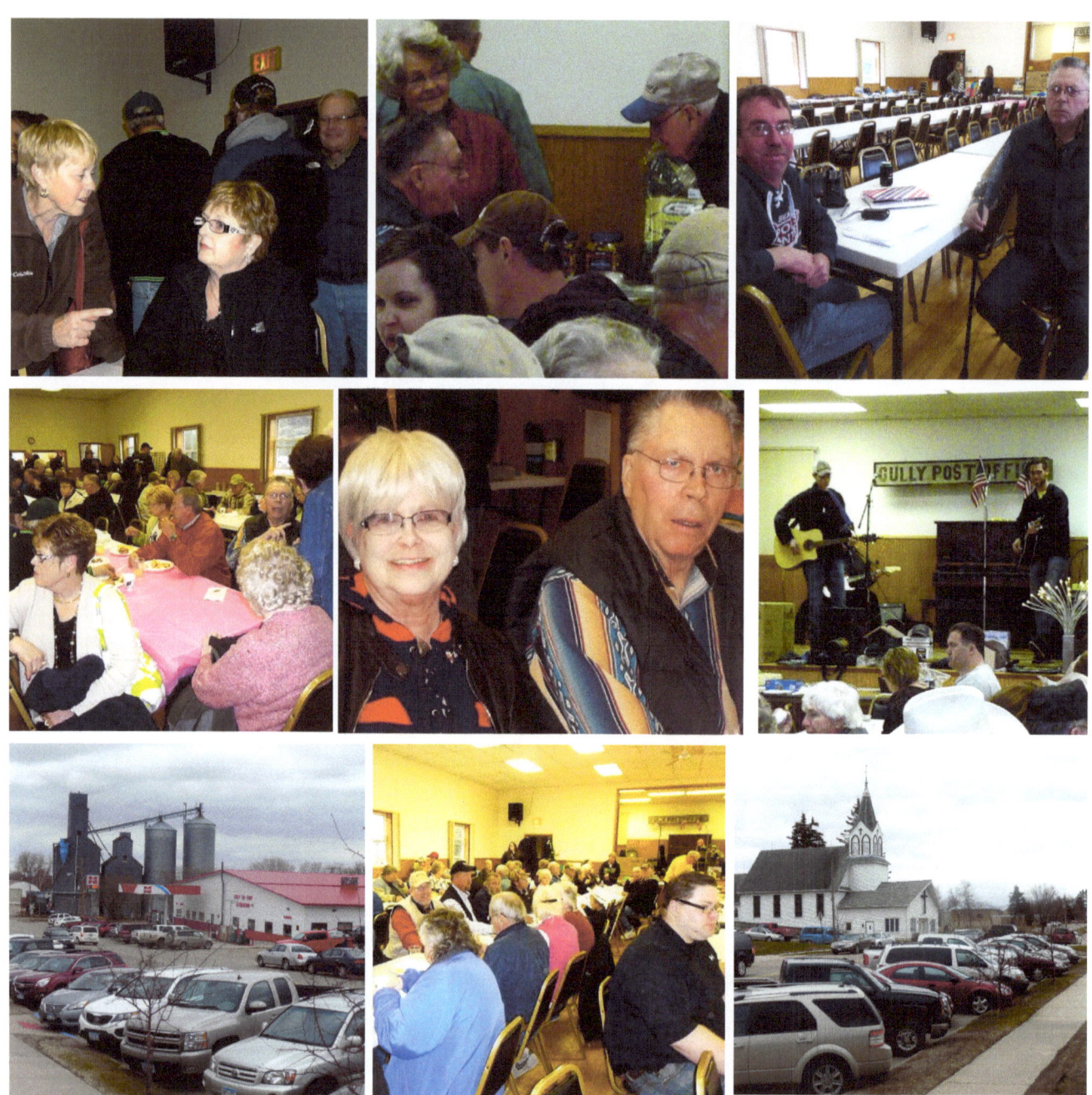

Benefit | Gully, MN | 4:30 - 8:30 P.M. | May 5, 2014

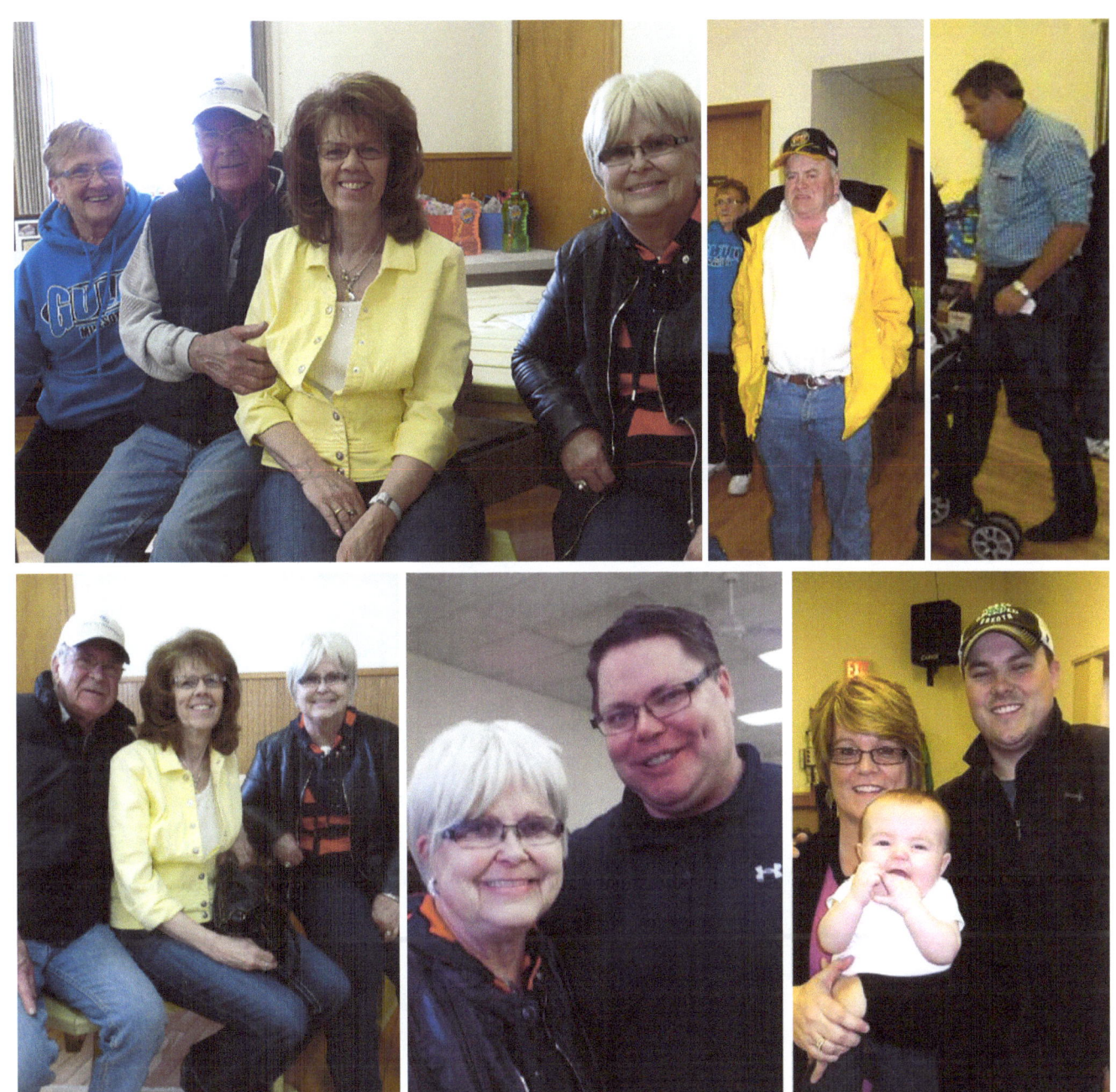

Benefit | Gully, MN | 4:30 - 8:30 P.M. | May 5, 2014

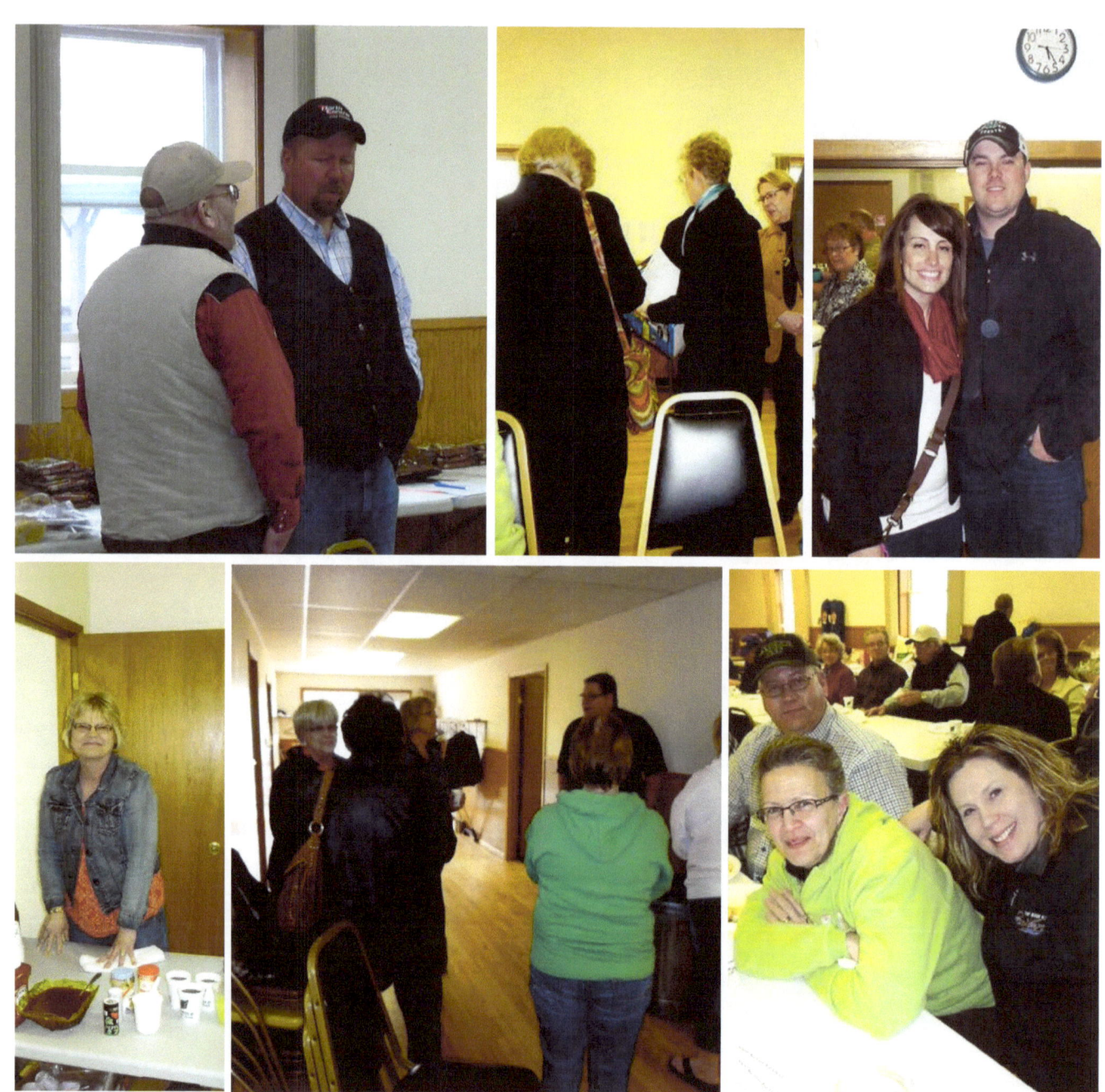

Benefit | Gully, MN | 4:30 - 8:30 P.M. | May 5, 2014

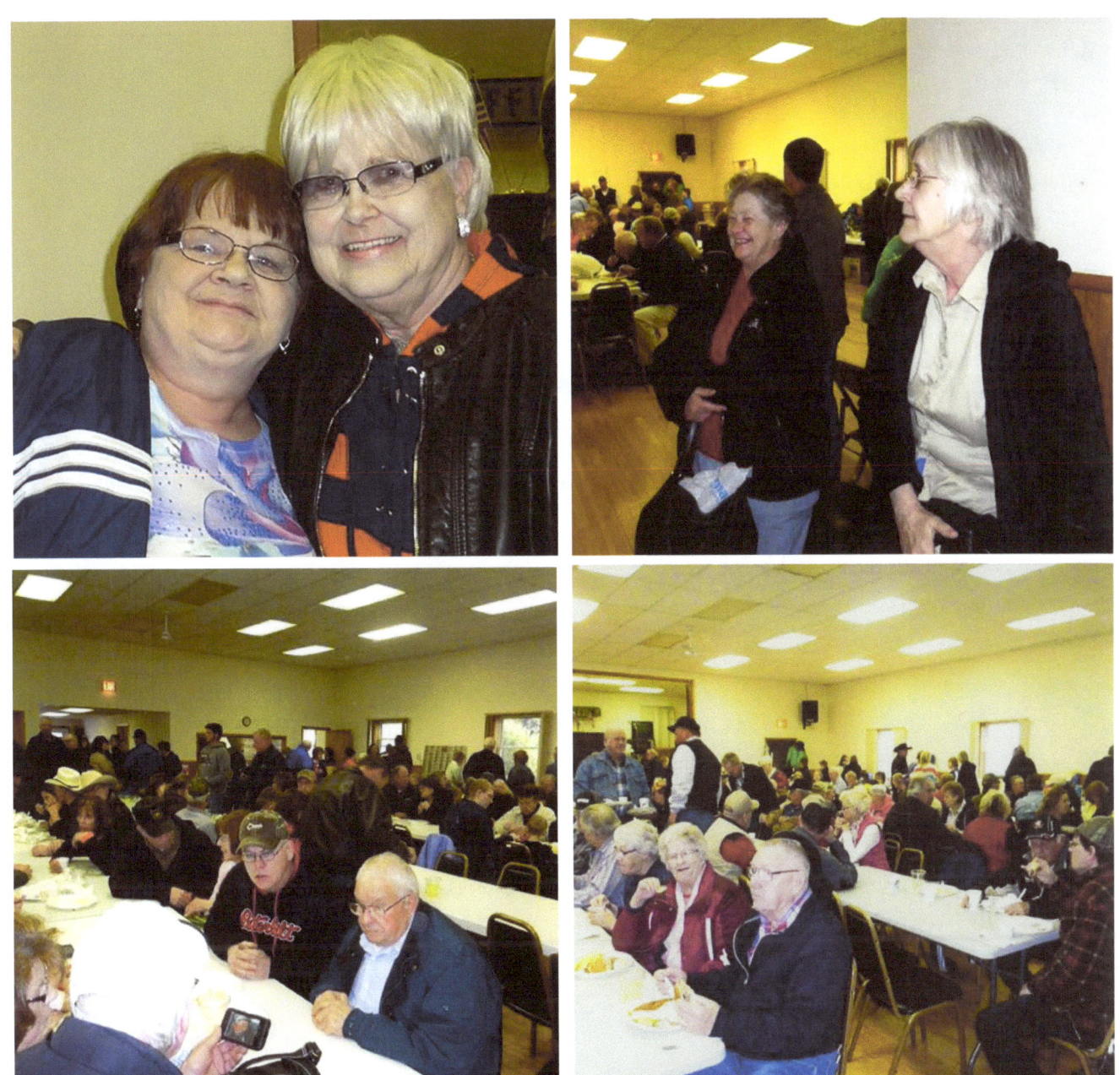

Benefit | Gully, MN | 4:30 - 8:30 P.M. | May 5, 2014

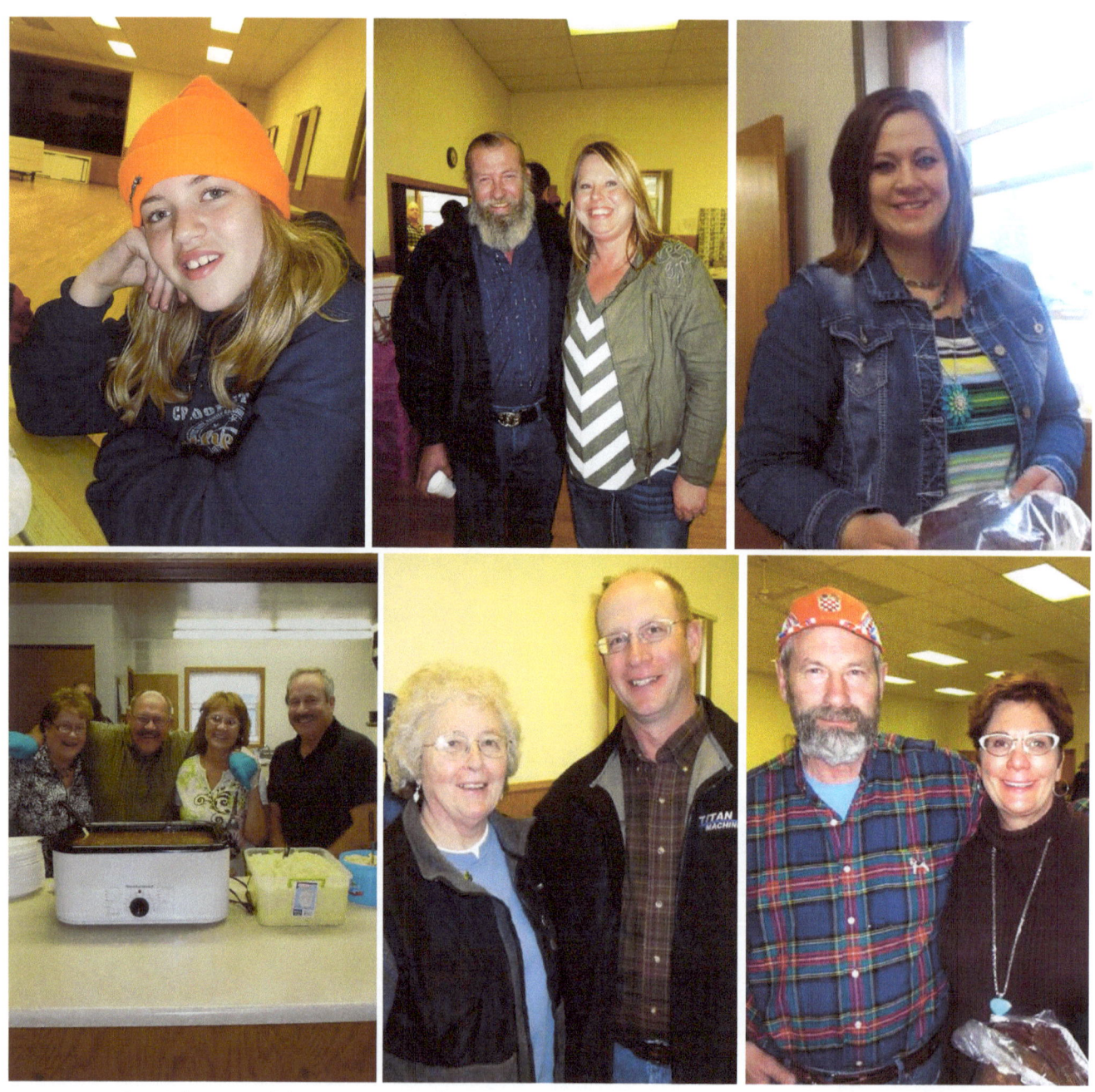

Benefit | Gully, MN | 4:30 - 8:30 P.M. | May 5, 2014

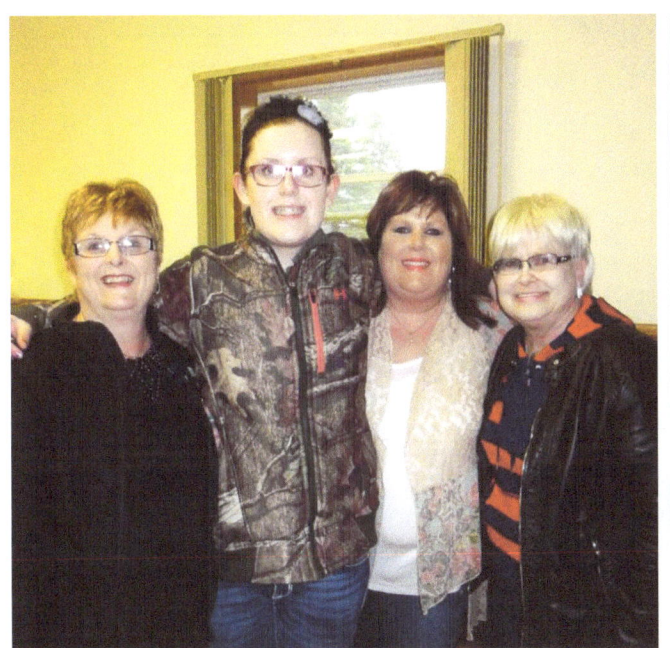

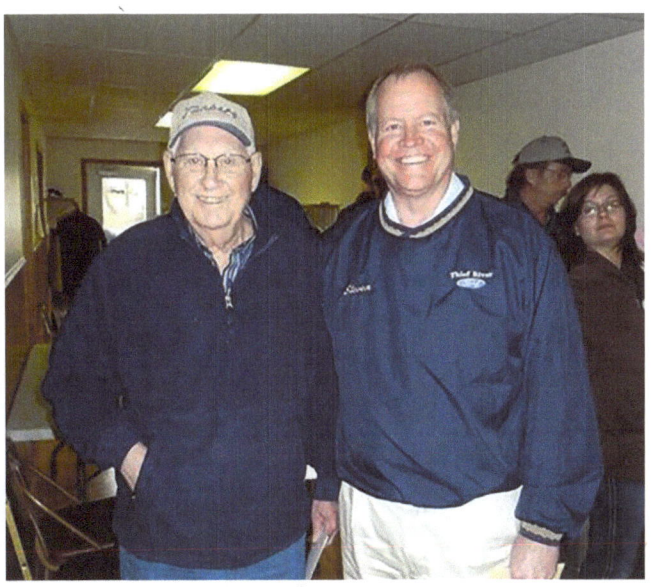

Ford Boys

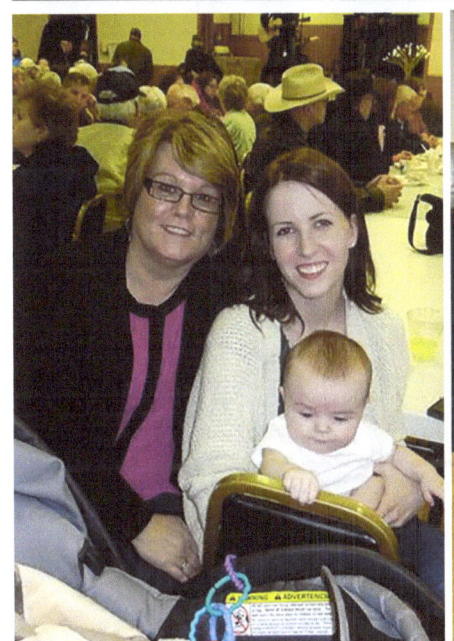

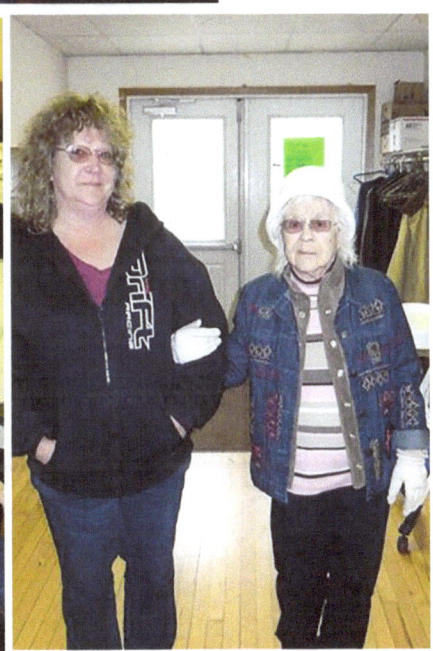

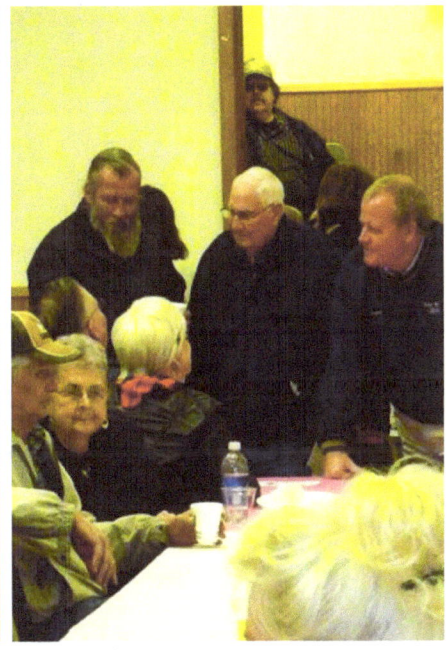

Benefit | Gully, MN | 4:30 - 8:30 P.M. | May 5, 2014

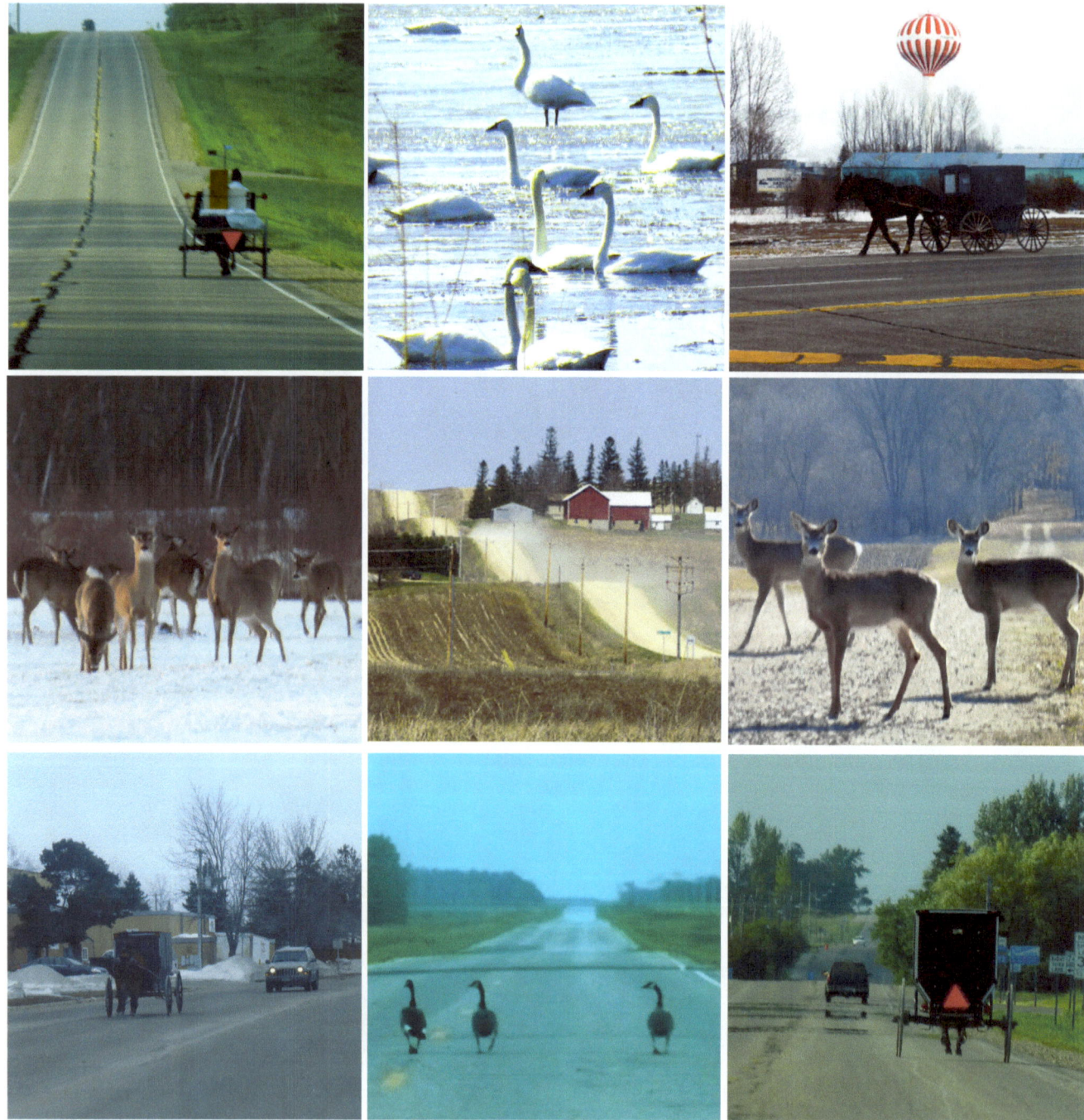

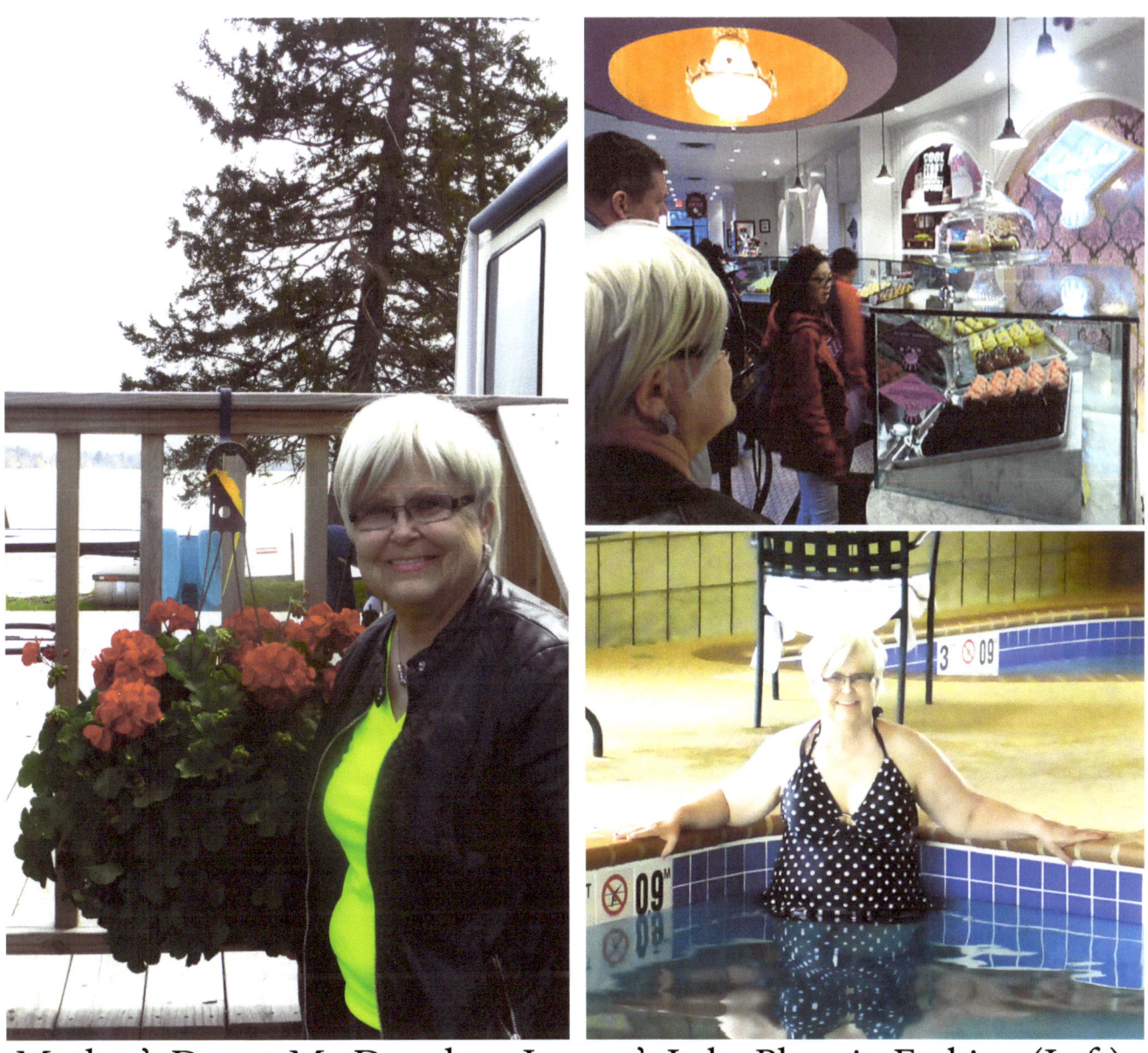

Mother's Day at My Daughter Joanne's Lake Place in Erskine (Left).
Cupcakes at Nadia Cakes in Maple Grove (Top-Right).
Exercising in Pool in Thief River Falls (Bottom-Right).

Skin Care

A few skin-care options were regularly recommended at the Mayo Clinic to prevent and treat radiation burns. These are excellent products, whether you use them for treating burns or day-to-day skin care. All are available most anywhere, including Wal-Mart. The daily routine for me was to apply Vanicream to the area being radiated at least three times a day during radiation treatments. Applying Vanicream minimized any burning until the highly-concentrated radiation treatments at the end of my radiation treatments, with a minimal sunburn and peeling of the skin, which is treated with diluted white vinegar.

Vanicream is made only about a ten minute drive from the Mayo Clinic in the town of Stewartville. Vanicream is all natural.

Aquaphor is a Vaseline/petroleum-based product. One of the nurse practitioners who I met with told how she accidentally scalded her arm with boiling water, applied Aquaphor, and her skin was back to normal a few hours later.

White vinegar diluted with water, applied with a wet wash cloth was also highly recommended for any burning, irritation, or redness caused by radiation.

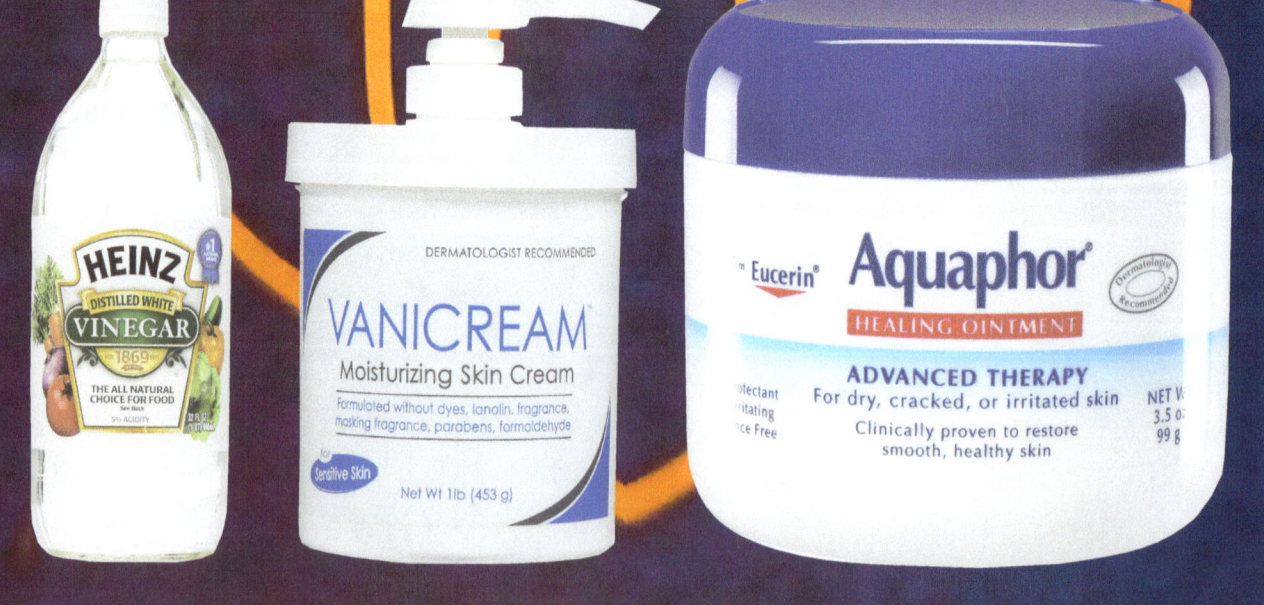

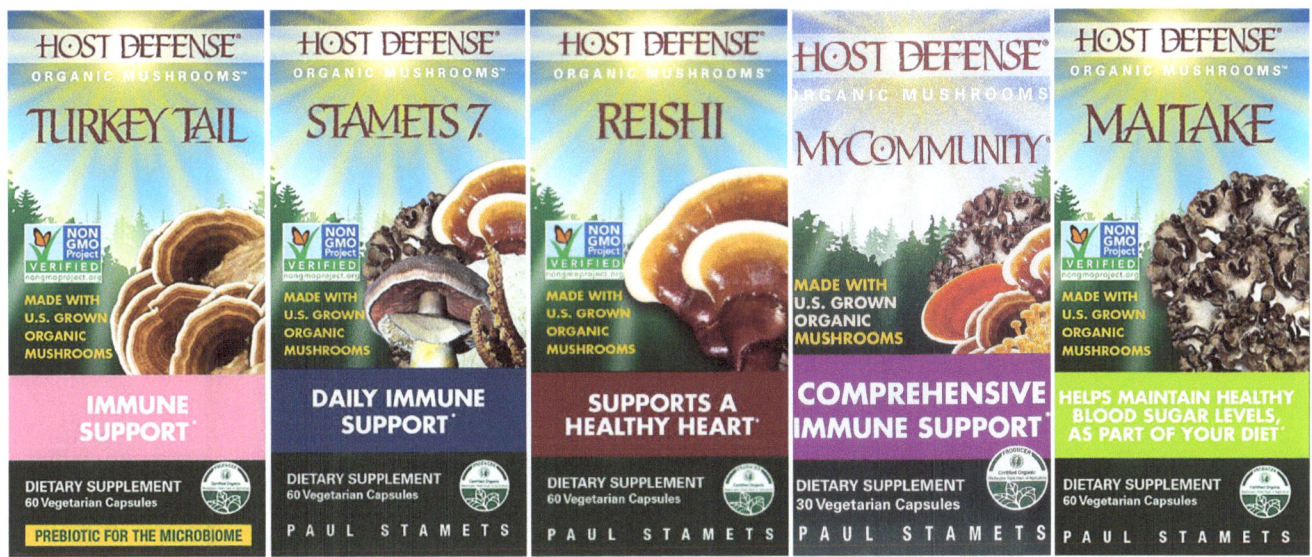

I take an alternative medication for my immune system. It is called Host Defense Organic Mushrooms. I believe that they have made it easier for me to get through the treatments.

Not a substitute for Western Medicine, rather these mushrooms are a supplement to support your body's natural immunity. Throughout my chemotherapy and radiation treatments, Mayo Clinic doctors and nurses were surprised at how good my overall health and blood levels were, when so many patients have their treatments interrupted due to low blood levels.

These mushrooms originate in old-growth forests and high-up in trees in the Pacific Northwest. The mushrooms are for folks who are interested in natural homeopathic, alternative, and preventative medicines. If they interest you, look-up Paul Stamets TEDMED speech "Mushroom Science No Trace of Cancer" online of his mother taking Turkey Tail Mushrooms to cure her Stage 4 Breast Cancer.

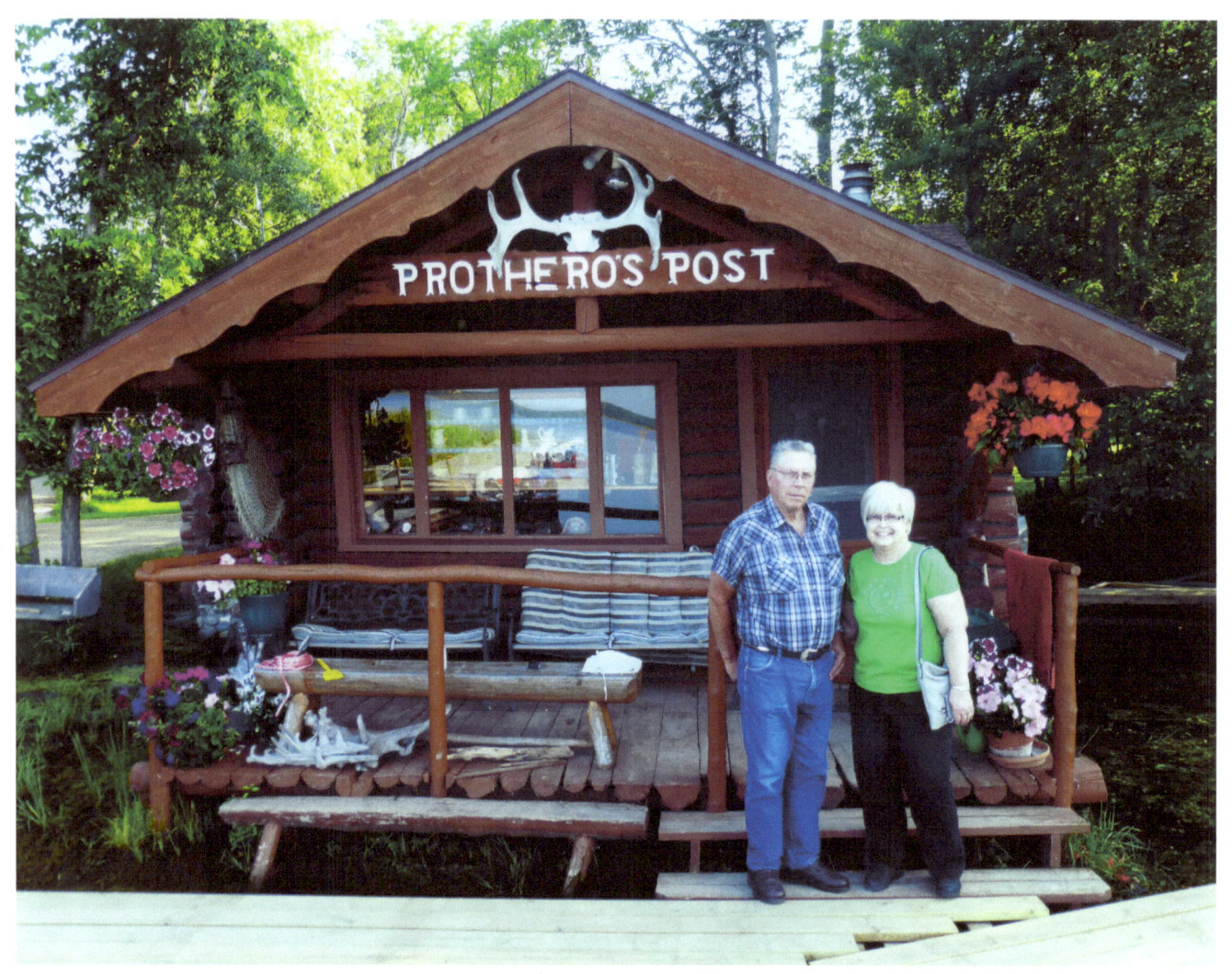

Minnesota's Northwest Angle
August 2014
Following Chemotherapy & Radiation Treatments.
Northernmost Point in Lower 48 States.
North of the 49TH Parallel.

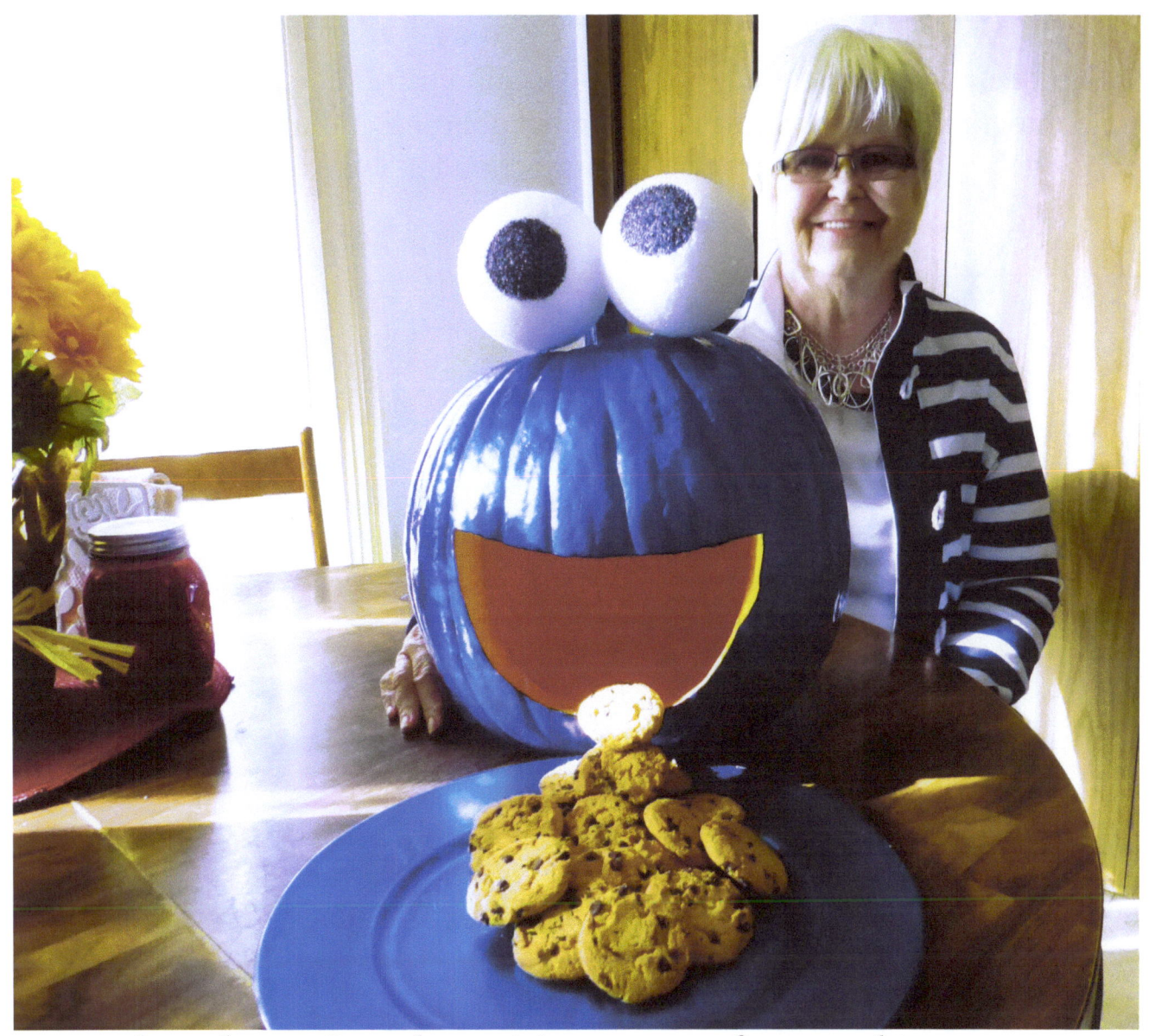

Made this Cookie Monster for a dinner we
had at church before Halloween.
It was a hit with the kids!

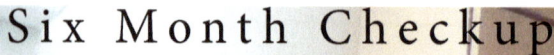

Six Month Checkup

Great news. Six months after my last radiation treatment. After a thorough mammogram, a doctor gave me a clean bill of health and told me that I do not need another mammogram for a year.

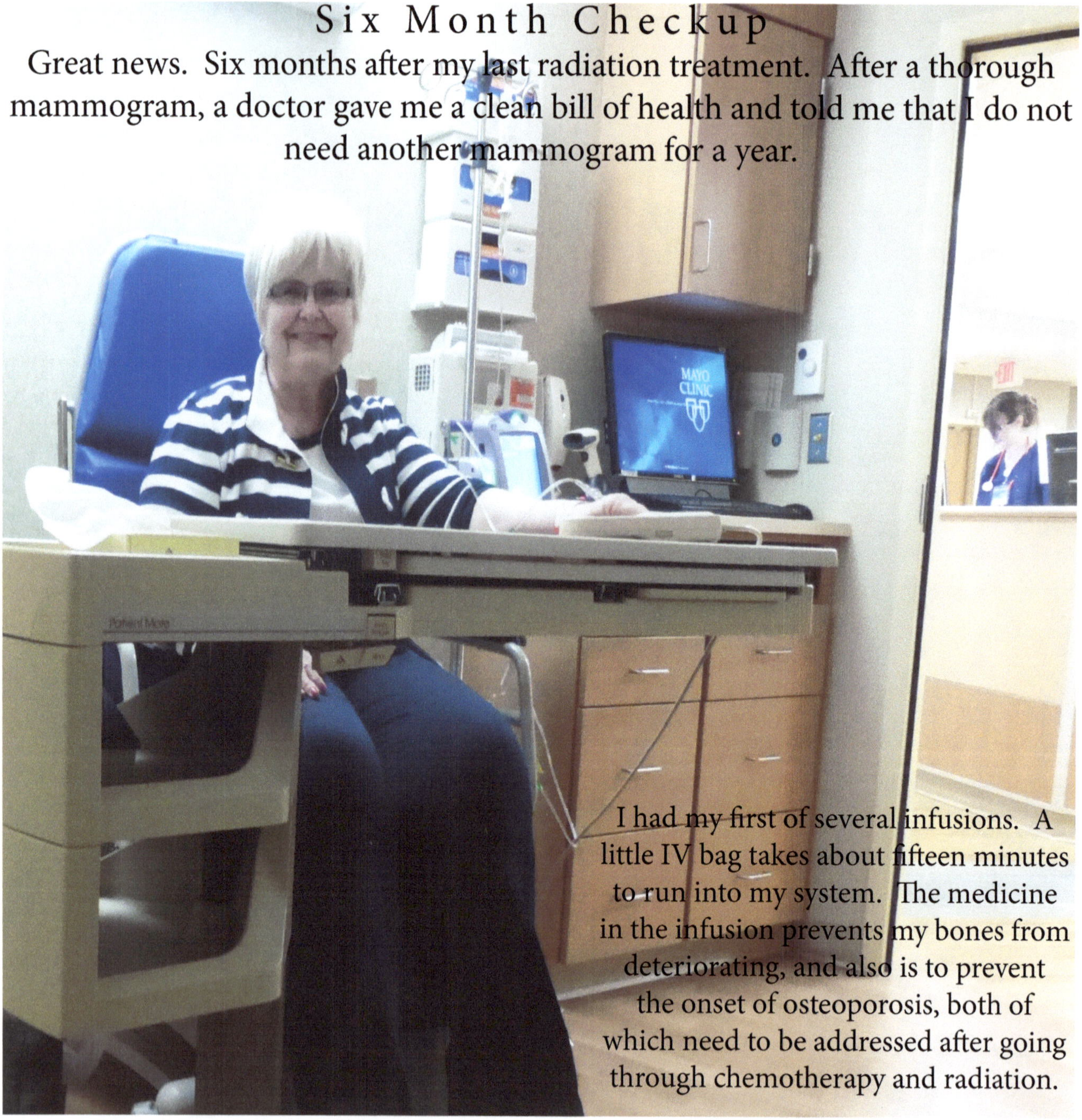

I had my first of several infusions. A little IV bag takes about fifteen minutes to run into my system. The medicine in the infusion prevents my bones from deteriorating, and also is to prevent the onset of osteoporosis, both of which need to be addressed after going through chemotherapy and radiation.

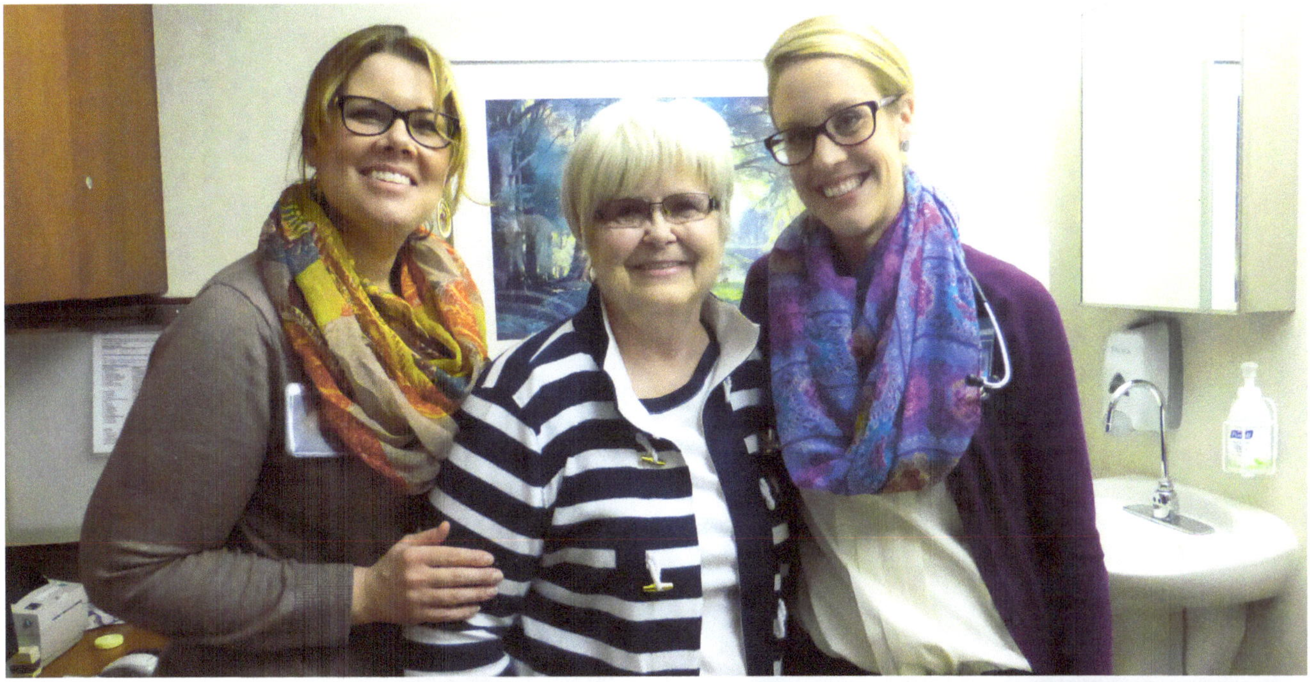

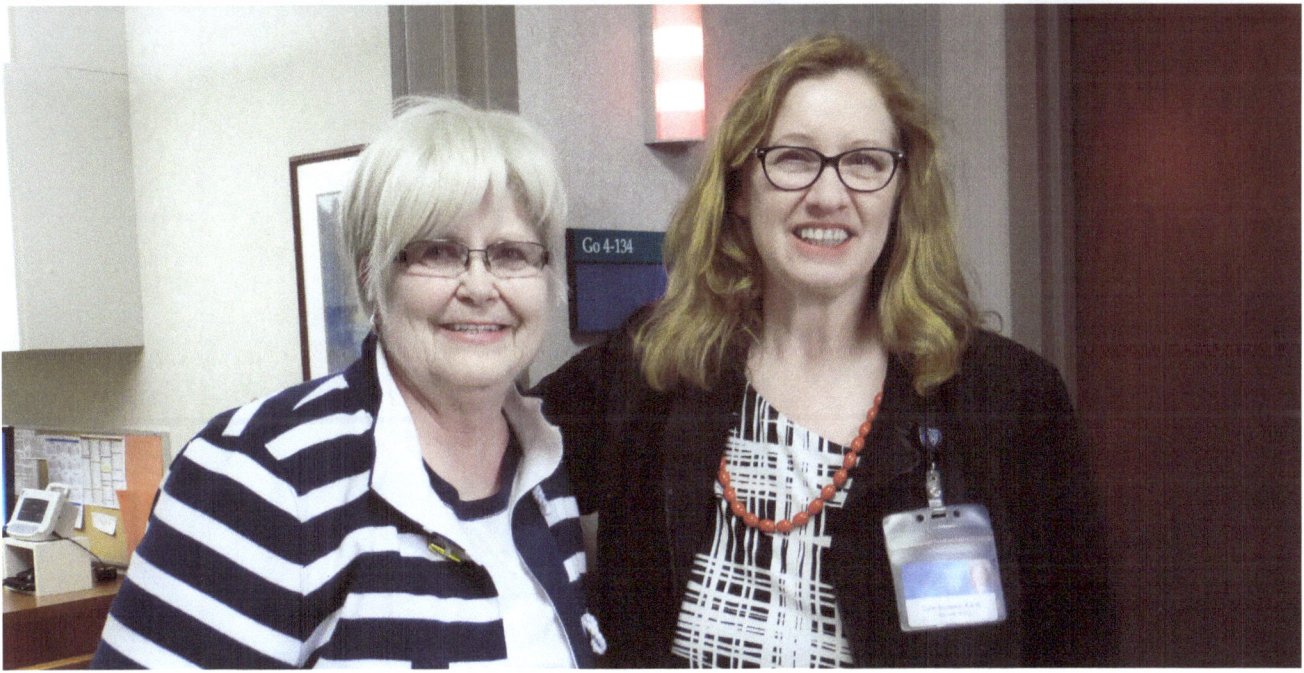

Last fall my cholesterol was high at 244 points. After one month, my cholesterol dropped to 166. I got my cholesterol down 78 points. A big reason for this positive change was because of going on a slow-carbohydrate, bean-based diet as outlined in Timothy Ferriss's book, "The 4-Hour Body."

The slow-carb bean diet consists of beans, lentils, vegetables, and non-processed meat. You can eat as much of these foods as you wish. One day a week, you are entitled to a "cheat day," where you can eat whatever foods your heart desires, including junk foods. This "cheat day" will not negatively effect your diet.

I also walked twice a day, lost weight, and felt good.

That month, I also started taking a prescribed cholesterol pill. My physician was amazed at how well I had done, telling me to "just keep it up."

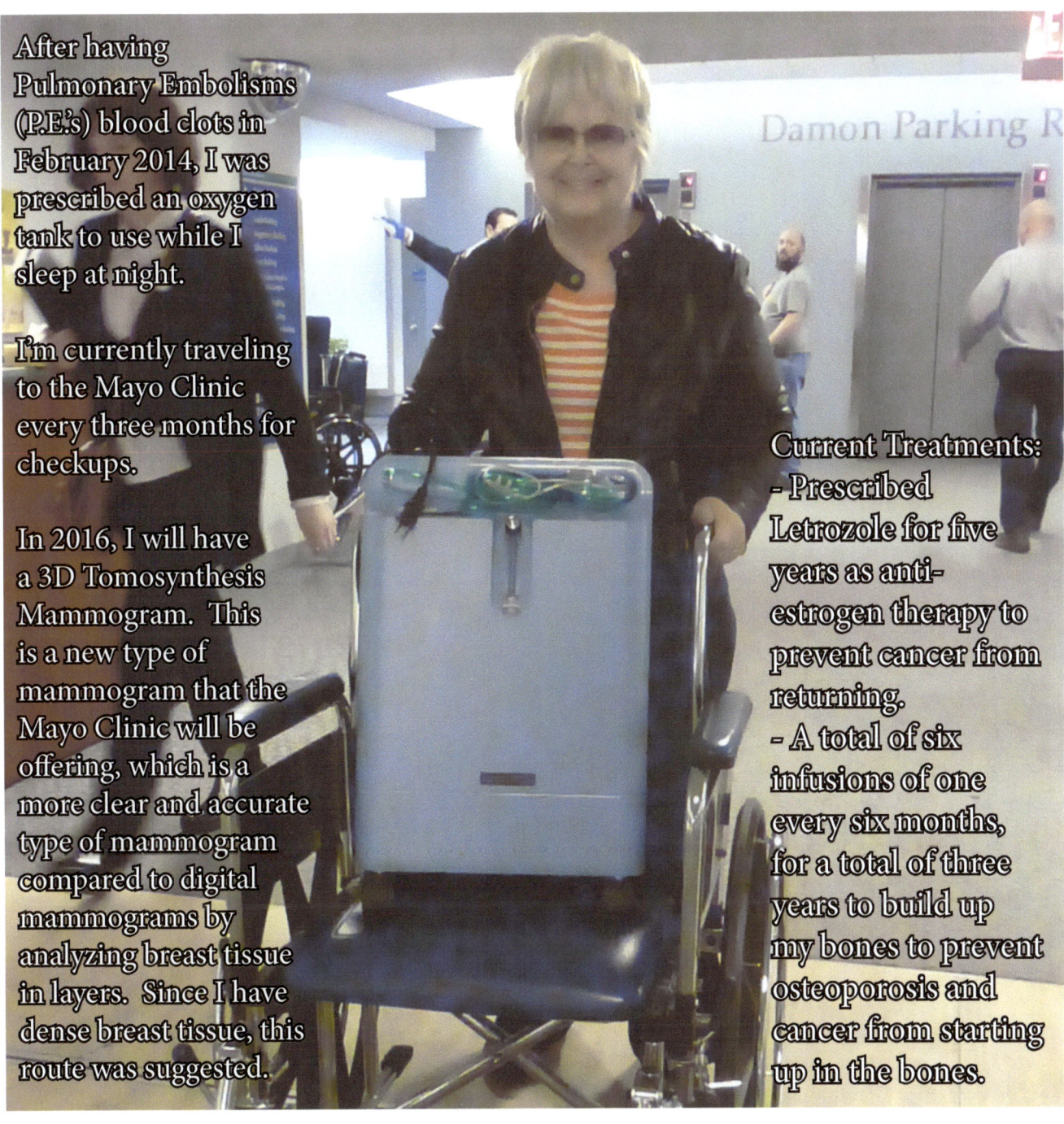

After having Pulmonary Embolisms (P.E.'s) blood clots in February 2014, I was prescribed an oxygen tank to use while I sleep at night.

I'm currently traveling to the Mayo Clinic every three months for checkups.

In 2016, I will have a 3D Tomosynthesis Mammogram. This is a new type of mammogram that the Mayo Clinic will be offering, which is a more clear and accurate type of mammogram compared to digital mammograms by analyzing breast tissue in layers. Since I have dense breast tissue, this route was suggested.

Current Treatments:
- Prescribed Letrozole for five years as anti-estrogen therapy to prevent cancer from returning.
- A total of six infusions of one every six months, for a total of three years to build up my bones to prevent osteoporosis and cancer from starting up in the bones.

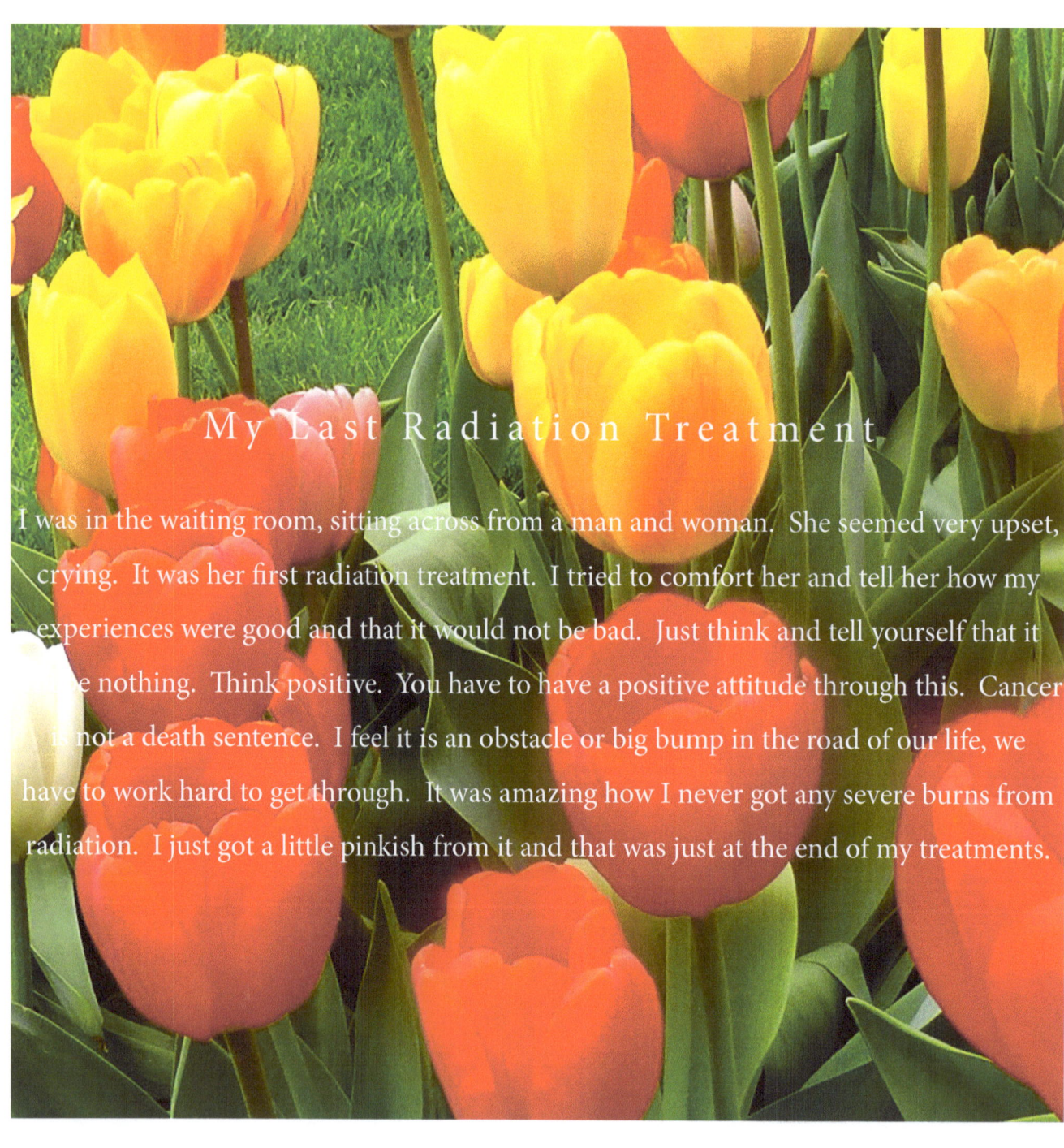

My Last Radiation Treatment

I was in the waiting room, sitting across from a man and woman. She seemed very upset, crying. It was her first radiation treatment. I tried to comfort her and tell her how my experiences were good and that it would not be bad. Just think and tell yourself that it be nothing. Think positive. You have to have a positive attitude through this. Cancer is not a death sentence. I feel it is an obstacle or big bump in the road of our life, we have to work hard to get through. It was amazing how I never got any severe burns from radiation. I just got a little pinkish from it and that was just at the end of my treatments.